Genitourinary

Genitourinary Radiology Cases

Mark E. Lockhart, MD, MPH
Professor of Radiology
Chief of Body Imaging and Genitourinary Radiology
University of Alabama at Birmingham School of Medicine
Birmingham, Alabama

Rupan Sanyal, MD
Assistant Professor of Radiology
Division of Body Imaging
University of Alabama at Birmingham School of Medicine
Birmingham, Alabama

OXFORD
UNIVERSITY PRESS

OXFORD
UNIVERSITY PRESS

Oxford University Press is a department of the University of
Oxford. It furthers the University's objective of excellence in research,
scholarship, and education by publishing worldwide.

Oxford   New York
Auckland   Cape Town   Dar es Salaam   Hong Kong   Karachi
Kuala Lumpur   Madrid   Melbourne   Mexico City   Nairobi
New Delhi   Shanghai   Taipei   Toronto

With offices in
Argentina   Austria   Brazil   Chile   Czech Republic   France   Greece
Guatemala   Hungary   Italy   Japan   Poland   Portugal   Singapore
South Korea   Switzerland   Thailand   Turkey   Ukraine   Vietnam

Oxford is a registered trademark of Oxford University Press
in the UK and certain other countries.

Published in the United States of America by
Oxford University Press
198 Madison Avenue, New York, NY 10016

© Oxford University Press 2014

Library of Congress Cataloging-in-Publication Data
Lockhart, Mark E., author.
Genitourinary radiology cases / Mark E. Lockhart, Rupan Sanyal.
    p. ; cm. —(Cases in radiology)
Includes bibliographical references and index.
ISBN 978–0–19–997574–7 (alk. paper)
I. Sanyal, Rupan, author.   II. Title.   III. Series: Cases in radiology.
[DNLM: 1. Female Urogenital Diseases—diagnosis—Case Reports.   2. Male Urogenital Diseases—
diagnosis—Case Reports.   3. Diagnostic Imaging—Case Reports.   4. Urogenital Neoplasms—
diagnosis—Case Reports.   WJ 141]
RC874
616.6′0754—dc23   2014007572

9 8 7 6 5 4 3 2 1
Printed in China
on acid-free paper

To my wife, Poonam, and my parents, for their love and support.

Rupan Sanyal

To my parents, my wife, and my children for their constant love and support.

Mark Lockhart

Acknowledgments

The Publisher thanks the following for their time and advice:

Mark Anderson, University of Virginia
Sanjeev Bhalla, Mallinckrodt Institute of Radiology, Washington University
Michael Bruno, Penn State Hershey Medical Center
Melissa Rosado de Christenson, St. Luke's Hospital of Kansas City
Rihan Khan, University of Arizona
Angela Levy, Georgetown University
Alexander Mamourian, University of Pennsylvania
Stacy Smith, Brigham and Women's Hospital

Preface

Education comes in many forms, and no two people learn in exactly the same way. In the practice of medicine, physicians have long been trained by a combination of didactic teaching, case-based learning, and apprenticeship during the performance of clinical care. While didactic teaching promotes passive learning, a case-based approach is more interactive and promotes active learning.

This inaugural edition of *Genitourinary Cases* is a collection of 129 individual examples of disease processes that affect a wide range of systems, with a focus on genitourinary imaging findings. As imagers, we have all experienced the discomfort that can arise as we face a case that fills us with uncertainty. It is in these moments that a great deal of learning can occur. The variety of cases presented will endeavor to cover the essentials of genitourinary radiology from the kidneys, ureters, bladder, adrenals, and retroperitoneum to the reproductive structures in a systematic grouping of pathology by general location. We hope that this will allow the reader to easily return to cases in the future, rather than serving as a singular opportunity to learn. Similarly, a list of diagnoses is provided to allow the reader to later refer back directly to a case without a broad search through the book.

A subspecialty such as radiology, which primarily deals with images, is particularly conducive to case-based learning. In this image-rich book, we have focused on the radiologic features and have tried to emphasize the differential diagnosis and practical teaching points for each case. We hope that this book will help the reader to identify and differentiate between the imaging appearances of various genitourinary diagnoses.

Contents

Section I Kidney

History

▶ 63-year-old man with weight loss

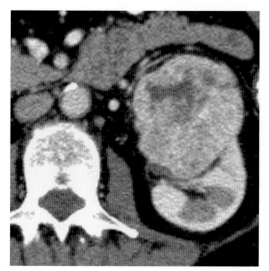

Figure 1.1

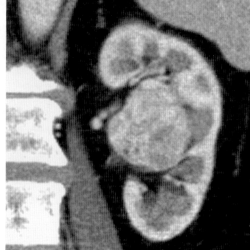

Figure 1.2

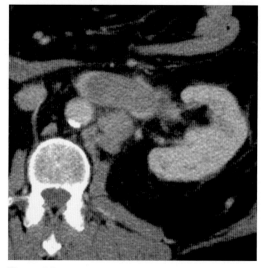

Figure 1.3

Case 1 Renal Cell Carcinoma: Clear Cell Subtype

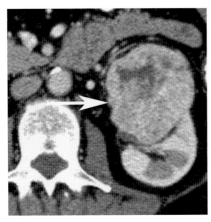 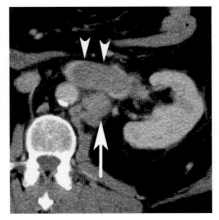

Figure 1.4   **Figure 1.5**

Findings

▸ Arterial-phase axial and coronal CT images (Figures 1.1 and 1.2) show a well-demarcated, avidly enhancing, heterogeneous, exophytic, cortical left renal mass (arrow in Figure 1.4).

▸ Portal venous-phase CT image (Figure 1.3) shows filling defect in the left renal vein (arrowheads in Figure 1.5); periaortic lymphadenopathy is present (arrow in Figure 1.5)

Differential Diagnosis

▸ Differential diagnosis of a renal mass includes renal cell carcinoma (RCC), transitional cell carcinoma (TCC), lymphoma, and oncocytoma. Renal TCCs are infiltrative, hypoenhancing, centrally located, noncontour-deforming masses and can be excluded. Renal lymphoma can present as a solitary renal mass but are hypoenhancing lesions. Oncocytomas are benign, well-demarcated, cortical lesions often indistinguishable from RCCs. Vascular invasion and adenopathy exclude oncocytoma. The well-defined, hyperenhancing, heterogeneous, exophytic cortical lesion seen here is consistent with RCC. The heterogeneous hyperenhancement favors clear cell subtype. Filling defect in the renal vein represents tumor thrombus, and the periaortic lymphadenopathy is consistent with nodal metastasis (stage T3a, N1, see below).

Teaching Points

▸ Histologic subtypes of RCC include clear cell or conventional carcinoma (80%), papillary carcinoma (15%), chromophobe carcinoma (5%), collecting duct carcinoma (1%), and unclassified (4%).

▸ Clear cell RCC has more avid and heterogeneous enhancement compared with papillary and chromophobe subtypes.

▸ According to the American Joint Committee on Cancer (AJCC) staging of RCC (2010), T1 is tumor <7 cm limited to kidney, T2 is tumor ≥7 cm limited to kidney, T3a is tumor extension into renal vein or perinephric fat, T3b is extension into inferior vena cava (IVC) below diaphragm, T3c is extension into IVC above diaphragm, and T4 is tumor extension beyond Gerota's fascia. Lymph nodal metastasis is N1 and distant metastasis is M1.

▸ Identifying extent of tumor invasion into the renal vein/IVC has significant implications on staging and surgery. Depending on level of thrombus, an abdominothoracic incision or cardiac bypass may be needed.

Management

▸ Partial or radical nephrectomy; systemic therapy for metastatic disease

Further Reading
Ng CS, Wood CG, Silverman PM, Tannir NM, Tamboli P, Sandler CM. Renal cell carcinoma: diagnosis, staging, and surveillance. *AJR Am J Roentgenol.* 2008;191(4):1220–1232.

History

▶ 71-year-old male with hematuria

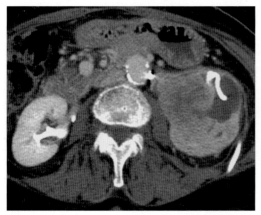

Figure 2.1

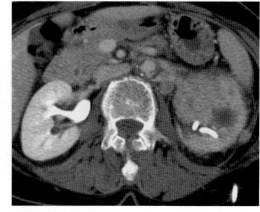

Figure 2.2

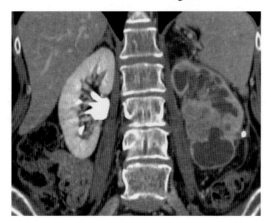

Figure 2.3

Case 2   Renal Pelvic Transitional Cell Carcinoma

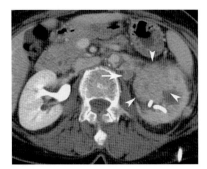

Figure 2.4

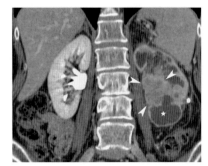

Figure 2.5

Findings

▸ Axial and coronal contrast-enhanced CT urogram images (Figures 2.1, 2.2 and 2.3) show a large, ill-defined, central hypoenhancing left renal lesion (arrowheads in Figures 2.4 and 2.5). The lesion has indistinct margins and infiltrates the renal parenchyma. It causes obstruction and dilation of multiple calyces (asterisk in Figure 2.5). Renal hilar lymphadenopathy is present (arrow in Figure 2.4). A pigtail catheter has been placed in a dilated calyx.

Differential Diagnosis

▸ Differential diagnosis of a solid enhancing renal mass includes renal cell carcinoma (RCC), transitional cell carcinoma (TCC), and lymphoma. The mass is hypoenhancing, infiltrating, centrally located in the kidney and maintains the reniform shape. These characteristics are typical of a renal pelvic TCC. RCCs are more common but have a cortical location, distinct margins, distort the renal contour, and are usually hyperenhancing. Renal lymphoma can present as a hypoenhancing perinephric mass, solitary or multifocal parenchymal lesions, or diffuse nephromegaly. Presence of lymphadenopathy helps identify renal lymphoma. It is important to identify renal TCC on imaging as it is treated with nephroureterectomy. Partial or radical nephrectomy is used for RCC and chemotherapy for lymphoma.

Teaching Points

▸ Approximately 15% of renal tumors are renal pelvic TCCs.
▸ There is a male preponderance with a peak incidence in the seventh decade.
▸ TCC is often multifocal, and approximately 30%–50% of patients with upper tract TCC develop bladder TCC.
▸ Renal TCCs arise from the renal pelvis/collecting system and infiltrate into the parenchyma. The reniform shape of the kidney is maintained on imaging.
▸ Upper tract TCCs spread by direct invasion and lymphatic spread.
▸ Lymph nodal metastasis has poor prognosis and is considered stage IV disease.

Management

▸ Nephroureterectomy and/or systemic therapy

Further Reading

Vikram R, Sandler CM, Ng CS. Imaging and staging of transitional cell carcinoma: part 2, upper urinary tract. *AJR Am J Roentgenol.* 2009;192(6):1488–1493.

History

▶ 60-year-old man with weight loss and flank pain (Figure 3.1; follow-up CT images were obtained after 4 months Figure 3.2)

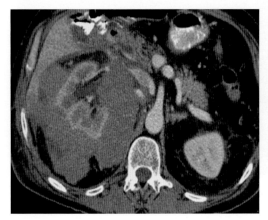

Figure 3.1

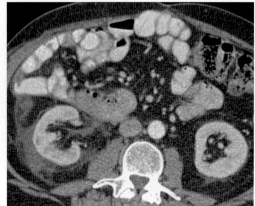

Figure 3.2

Case 3 Perinephric Lymphoma

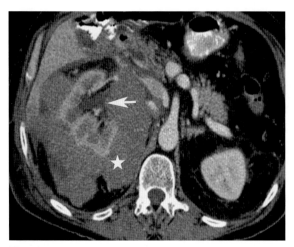

Figure 3.3

Findings

▶ Contrast-enhanced CT (Figure 3.1) shows a large, homogeneous, mildly enhancing perinephric mass encasing the right kidney (asterisk in Figure 3.3). The large perinephric component displaces and distorts the renal parenchyma and extends to the renal hilum (arrow in Figure 3.3).
▶ Follow-up CT after chemotherapy reveals significant interval reduction with small residual perinephric soft tissue (Figure 3.2).

Differential Diagnosis

▶ Differential diagnosis of perinephric soft tissue includes lymphoma, sarcoma, retroperitoneal fibrosis, and perinephric hematoma. Perinephric hematomas can be identified by drop in hematocrit, history of trauma, or biopsy and lack of enhancement. Although retroperitoneal fibrosis can present as perinephric soft tissue, it usually affects the periaortic lower retroperitoneum and is less bulky. Retroperitoneal sarcomas show heterogeneous enhancement and do not typically have perinephric distribution. Bulky, homogeneously hypoenhancing perinephric soft tissue, as seen in this, case would favor lymphoma.

Teaching Points

▶ Renal lymphoma manifests as a solitary renal mass, multifocal/bilateral renal masses, perinephric masses, or diffuse nephromegaly.
▶ Perinephric lymphoma can occur from direct extension of retroperitoneal lymphadenopathy or transcapsular spread of parenchymal disease, or it can represent the only manifestation.
▶ Perirenal lymphoma can completely surround the kidney without functional impairment or parenchymal compression.
▶ Extension into the renal hilum may encase the renal vessels.
▶ Perinephric lymphoma is homogeneous and hypoenhancing on CT.

Management

▶ Percutaneous biopsy can confirm the diagnosis followed by appropriate chemotherapy.

Further Reading

Westphalen A, Yeh B, Qayyum A, Hari A, Coakley FV. Differential diagnosis of perinephric masses on CT and MRI. *AJR Am J Roentgenol.* 2004;183(6):1697–1702.

History

▶ 48-year-old male with weight loss

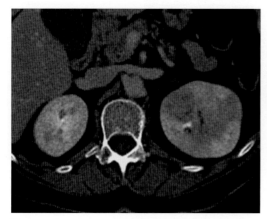

Figure 4.1

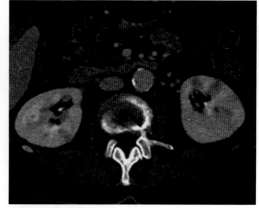

Figure 4.2

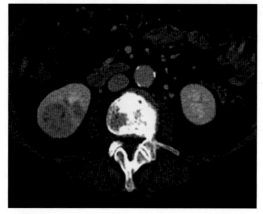

Figure 4.3

Case 4 Lymphoma: Multifocal Renal Masses

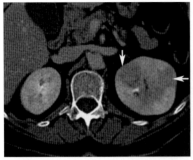

Figure 4.4

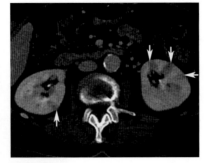

Figure 4.5

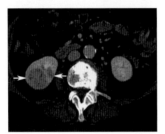

Figure 4.6

Findings

▸ Contrast-enhanced CT images (Figures 4.1, 4.2 and 4.3) show multiple, hypoenhancing, solid parenchymal masses in both kidneys (arrows in Figures 4.4, 4.5 and 4.6).

Differential Diagnosis

▸ Differential diagnosis for bilateral, multifocal, hypoenhancing, endophytic parenchymal masses includes lymphoma, metastases, and pyelonephritis. All three can have a similar imaging appearance. Concomitant lymphadenopathy and splenomegaly favor lymphoma. Renal metastases usually occur in the presence of extensive systemic metastases. Clinical presentation and urinalysis help identify pyelonephritis.

Teaching Points

▸ Kidneys do not contain lymphoid tissue, and primary renal lymphoma is rare.
▸ Renal involvement is due to extranodal spread of lymphoma. Renal involvement is present in one-third of cases on autopsy, although findings on imaging studies for staging are much less common. It occurs more commonly with non-Hodgkin disease than Hodgkin lymphoma.
▸ Renal lymphoma manifests as a solitary renal mass, multifocal/bilateral renal masses, perinephric masses, or diffuse nephromegaly. Multiple bilateral renal masses are the most common presentation, occurring in 40%–60% of patients.
▸ Renal lymphoma is usually accompanied by extra-renal disease in other organs and/or lymph nodes.
▸ On unenhanced CT imaging, renal lymphoma is iso- or hypodense to parenchyma. After contrast administration, lymphoma enhances less than the adjacent parenchyma and has a relatively homogeneous appearance.
▸ On ultrasound, renal lymphoma is hypoechoic to renal parenchyma and may simulate a cyst.

Management

▸ Renal lymphoma is treated with chemotherapy; most other renal neoplasms routinely undergo surgical resection without preoperative biopsy. If the diagnosis of lymphoma is in question on imaging, a biopsy may establish the diagnosis and guide appropriate chemotherapy.

Further Reading

Sheth S, Ali S, Fishman E. Imaging of renal lymphoma: patterns of disease with pathologic correlation. *Radiographics*. 2006;26(4):1151–1168.

History

▶ 23-year-old female with acute renal failure and abdominal pain (Figures 5.1 and 5.2); follow-up contrast-enhanced CT image after 3 months of therapy was obtained (Figure 5.3)

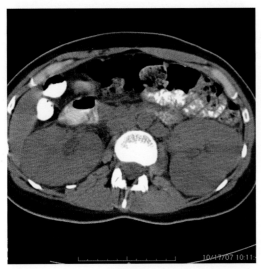

Figure 5.1

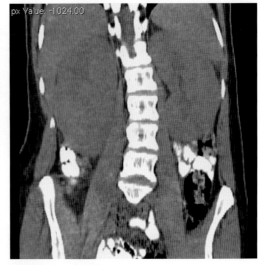

Figure 5.2

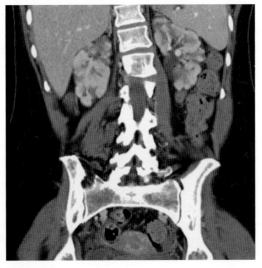

Figure 5.3

Case 5 Lymphoma with Nephromegaly

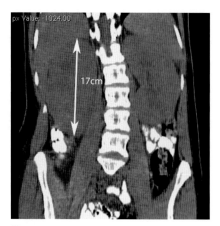

Figure 5.4

Findings

▶ Unenhanced CT images (5.1, 5.2, and 5.4) show massive smooth enlargement of both kidneys; no focal mass identified.

▶ Follow-up CT after 3 months of chemotherapy (Figure 5.3) shows significant reduction in renal size with extensive parenchymal scarring.

Differential Diagnosis

▶ Differential diagnosis for bilateral smooth renal enlargement includes diabetes, acute glomerulonephritis, autoimmune diseases such as systemic lupus erythematosus, polyarteritis nodosa, Wegener's granulomatosis, Henoch–Schönlein purpura, human immunodeficiency virus nephropathy, and neoplastic processes such as lymphoma and leukemia. The massive nephromegaly noted here is unusual for a benign process and favors lymphoma or leukemia.

Teaching Points

▶ Renal lymphoma manifests as a solitary renal mass, multifocal/bilateral renal masses, perinephric masses, or diffuse nephromegaly. Diffuse nephromegaly is the least common of these manifestations.

▶ Nephromegaly without distortion of the renal shape is caused by infiltration of the renal interstitium by lymphocytes.

▶ Diffuse nephromegaly is most commonly seen in Burkitt's lymphoma and may be part of disseminated disease or limited to the kidneys.

▶ Destruction of normal renal architecture by lymphoma in these patients can present as acute renal failure.

▶ Rapid reduction in renal size and improvement in renal function are seen after institution of chemotherapy for lymphoma.

Management

▶ Percutaneous biopsy is performed to confirm the diagnosis in cases indeterminate by imaging to guide appropriate chemotherapy.

Further Reading
Sheth S, Ali S, Fishman E. Imaging of renal lymphoma: patterns of disease with pathologic correlation. *Radiographics.* 2006;26(4):1151–1168.

History

► 60-year-old man with incidental renal mass

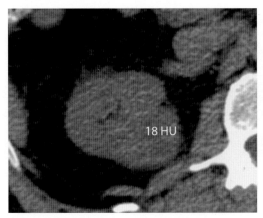

Figure 6.1

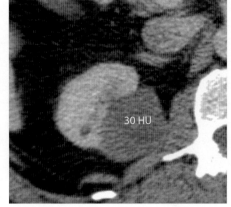

Figure 6.2

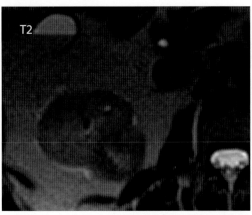

Figure 6.3

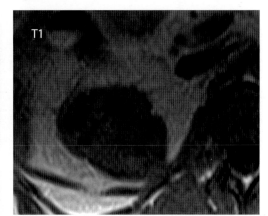

Figure 6.4

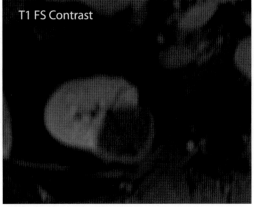

Figure 6.5

Case 6 Papillary Renal Cell Carcinoma

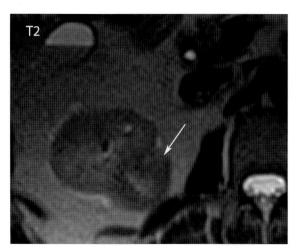

Figure 6.6

Findings

▸ Unenhanced and contrast-enhanced CT images show a homogeneous, mildly enhancing (enhancement by 12 HU) cortical neoplasm (Figures 6.1 and 6.2).

▸ On MRI, the mass is mildly hypointense to renal parenchyma on T2 imaging (Figures 6.3 and 6.6), isointense on T1 imaging (Figure 6.4), and enhances less than the parenchyma during nephrographic phase (Figure 6.5).

Differential Diagnosis

▸ Differential diagnosis for enhancing cortical renal neoplasm includes common subtypes of renal cell carcinomas (RCCs); clear cell, papillary, and chromophobe), benign oncocytomas, and lipid poor angiomyolipomas. Clear cell RCCs, oncocytomas, and lipid poor angiomyolipomas show avid contrast enhancement; chromophobe RCCs show moderate enhancement; and papillary RCCs show mild enhancement. Clear cell RCCs, chromophobe RCCs, and onchocytomas are usually hyper- or isointense to renal parenchyma on T2-weighted images, while papillary RCCs and lipid-poor angiomyolipomas are frequently hypointense on T2 imaging. Papillary RCCs and lipid-poor angiomyolipomas demonstrate homogeneous enhancement compared with heterogeneous enhancement of clear cell RCCs. In this patient, a T2 hypointense mass with mild homogeneous enhancement favors papillary RCC.

Teaching Points

▸ Papillary RCC is the second most common type of RCC (after clear cell) and accounts for 10%–15% of all RCCs.

▸ Bilateral and multifocal tumors are more common in papillary RCC than other RCC subtypes.

▸ Papillary RCCs are hypovascular compared with clear cell RCCs and show mild, homogeneous enhancement. Larger tumors show heterogeneity due to necrosis, hemorrhage, and calcification.

▸ They are often hypointense on T2-weighted imaging, which helps to differentiate them from more common clear cell RCCs.

▸ Papillary RCCs have better prognosis than clear cell RCCs (87% 5-year survival rate compared with 69%).

Management

▸ Localized papillary RCC is surgically resected. Metastatic disease is treated with systemic therapy.

Further Reading

Vikram R, Ng CS, Tamboli P, et al. Papillary renal cell carcinoma: radiologic-pathologic correlation and spectrum of disease. *Radiographics*. 2009;29(3):741–754.

History

▶ 55-year-old male with gross hematuria

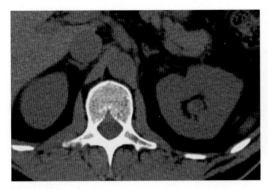

Figure 7.1

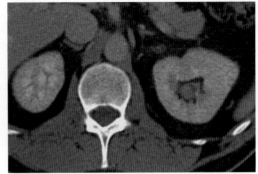

Figure 7.2

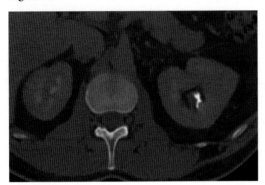

Figure 7.3

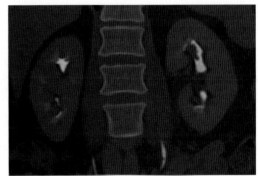

Figure 7.4

Case 7   Upper Tract Calyceal Transitional Cell Carcinoma

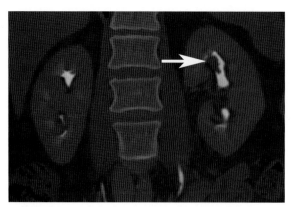

Figure 7.5

Findings

▶ Unenhanced (Figure 7.1), nephrographic (Figure 7.2), and delayed-phase CT images (Figures 7.3 and 7.4) show a small, mildly enhancing nodule in the upper collecting system (arrow in Figure 7.5). It is difficult to identify on the unenhanced CT and is best seen outlined by contrast in the collecting system on the excretory phase (bone window).

Differential Diagnosis

▶ Differential diagnosis of filling defect in the collecting system includes transitional cell carcinoma and blood clot. Blood clot can be excluded as they are high attenuation on unenhanced CT and do not enhance after contrast administration. Enhancement in the collecting system lesion noted here is consistent with a small upper tract transitional cell carcinoma (TCC). Large renal TCCs should be differentiated from renal cell carcinomas (RCCs). TCCs are hypoenhancing, infiltrative, centrally located in the kidney, and maintain the reniform shape. RCCs have a cortical location, distinct margins, distort the renal contour, and are usually hyperenhancing.

Teaching Points

▶ TCC involves the lining of the bladder, ureter, and collecting system in a ratio of 50:3:1.
▶ It can be multifocal, and 30%–50% of patients with upper tract tumor develop bladder tumor. Patients with bladder tumor have 2%–3% chance of developing upper tract tumor.
▶ Gross, painless hematuria is the most common clinical presentation of TCC.
▶ CT urography with excretory-phase imaging is recommended for evaluation of hematuria. Opacification of the collecting system on the excretory-phase allows detection of small TCCs.
▶ Upper tract TCCs are more aggressive than bladder tumors. They commonly spread by direct invasion and lymphatic route.
▶ Any lymph nodal metastasis is considered stage IV disease and has poor prognosis.

Management

▶ Nephroureterectomy

Further Reading

Vikram R, Sandler CM, Ng CS. Imaging and staging of transitional cell carcinoma: part 2, upper urinary tract. *AJR Am J Roentgenol.* 2009;192(6):1488–1493.

History

▶ 50-year-old man with incidental renal lesion

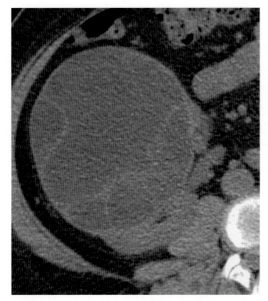

Figure 8.1

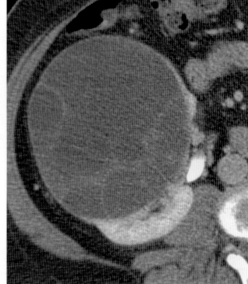

Figure 8.2

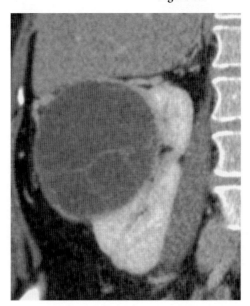

Figure 8.3

Case 8   Bosniak III Renal Cyst

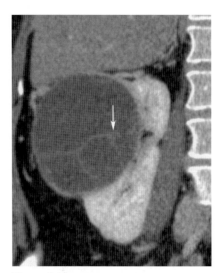

Figure 8.4

Findings

▶ Unenhanced (Figure 8.1) and contrast-enhanced CT images (Figures 8.2 and 8.3) show a large partially exophytic right renal cyst. Multiple mildly enhancing septa with areas of thickening and irregularity are present (arrow in Figure 8.4). Cyst wall thickening is also seen.

Differential Diagnosis

▶ Renal cysts are stratified on imaging according to the Bosniak classification. Bosniak IIF cysts may have minimally thick septa but no irregularity or measurable enhancement. Bosniak IV cysts have distinct enhancing soft tissue component independent of the wall or septa. In this patient, areas of irregular septal thickening and enhancement classify the lesion as a Bosniak III renal cyst. Bosniak III category lesions may include hemorrhagic or infected cysts, multilocular cystic nephroma, and cystic renal cell cancer.

Teaching Points

▶ The Bosniak classification is not a pathological classification of renal cysts but a CT-based imaging and clinical management system.
▶ Category I (simple cysts) and category II (mildly complex cysts that may have few hairline septa with perceivable but not measurable enhancement; fine or short segment calcification; or hyperdense cysts <3 cm) cysts are dismissed as benign.
▶ Category IIF cysts are thought to be benign but need to be followed to confirm stability. This includes cysts with multiple hairline septa; perceived but not measurable enhancement in smooth septa; minimal thickening of cyst wall or septa; thick calcification; and intrarenal hyperdense cysts >3 cm.
▶ Category III cysts have thick irregular or smooth wall or septa with measurable enhancement; 40%–60% of Bosniak III cysts are malignant, and surgical resection is needed in most cases.
▶ Category IV cysts have distinct enhancing soft tissue components and have a high likelihood of malignancy.
▶ Pitfalls when applying the Bosniak classification include pseudo enhancement in cysts (usually <2 cm) when surrounded by enhancing parenchyma and difficulty in detecting enhancement in heavily calcified lesions.

Management

▶ Surgical resection

Further Reading
Freire M, Remer EM. Clinical and radiologic features of cystic renal masses. *AJR Am J Roentgenol.* 2009;192(5):1367–1372.

Case 9

History

- 49-year-old man with right flank pain

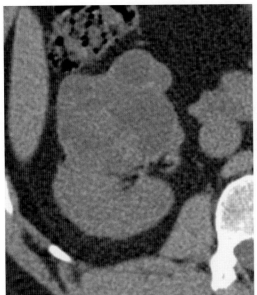

Figure 9.1

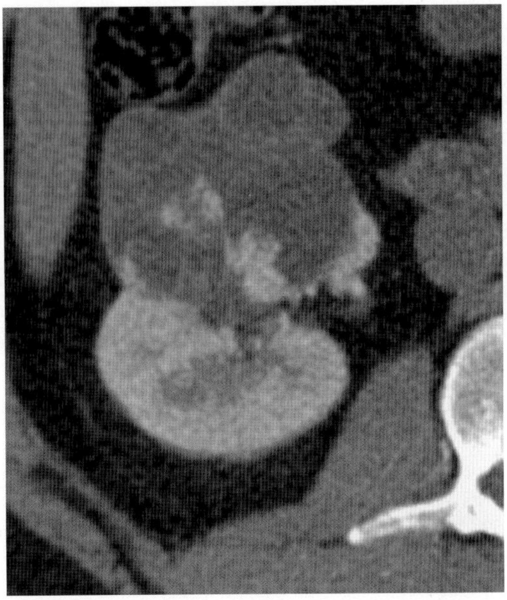

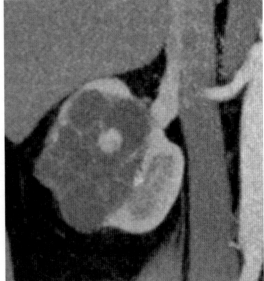

Figure 9.2

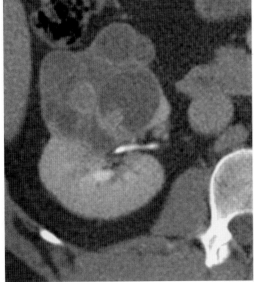

Figure 9.3

Figure 9.4

Case 9 Bosniak IV Renal Cyst

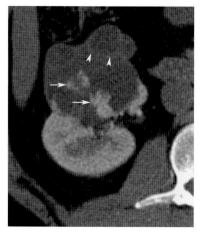 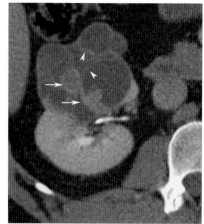

Figure 9.5   **Figure 9.6**

Findings

▶ Unenhanced (Figure 9.1), corticomedullary (Figures 9.2 and 9.4), and nephrographic -phase CT images (Figure 9.3) show a large, lobulated, partially exophytic right renal cyst with distinct enhancing soft tissue components (arrows in Figures 9.5 and 9.6) and multiple enhancing internal septations (arrowheads in Figures 9.5 and 9.6).

Differential Diagnosis

▶ Presence of enhancing nodular soft tissue component classifies this lesion as a malignant Bosniak IV cyst. Bosniak III cysts, which may or may not be malignant, can have enhancing septa but do not have enhancing soft tissue component, as in this patient.

Teaching Points

▶ The Bosniak classification of renal cysts is used to differentiate between surgical and nonsurgical cysts. Bosniak III and IV cysts are typically considered surgical lesions.

▶ Studies have shown that 95%–100% of Bosniak IV renal cysts are malignant.

▶ Bosniak IV cysts can have all features of Bosniak III cysts but have additional distinct enhancing soft tissue component independent of the wall or septa.

▶ Up to 15% of renal cell carcinomas (RCCs) have a cystic component. This includes RCCs with necrotic/hemorrhagic change and true cystic renal cell carcinoma (CRCC). True CRCCs do not have necrosis, differentiating them from conventional RCC with cystic appearance due to necrosis.

▶ CRCCs have better prognosis (87% 5-year survival) than conventional clear cell RCCs. The majority of CRCCs are stage I on detection.

▶ RCCs with cystic appearance due to necrosis have similar prognosis to solid RCCs.

Management

▶ Surgical resection

Further Reading
Israel GM, Bosniak MA. How I do it: evaluating renal masses. *Radiology.* 2005;236(2):441–450.

History

▶ 55-year-old female with incidental left renal lesion

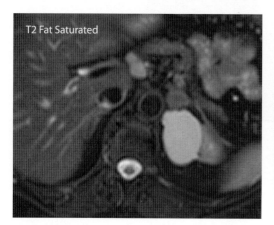

Figure 10.1

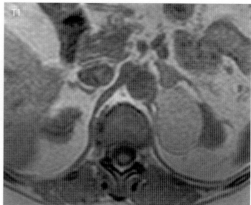

Figure 10.2

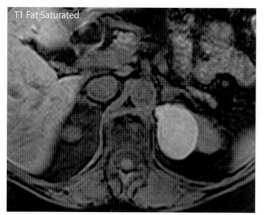

Figure 10.3

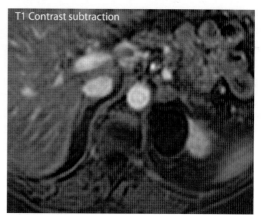

Figure 10.4

Case 10   Hemorrhagic Renal Cyst

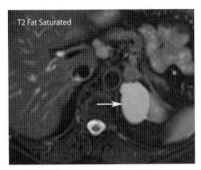 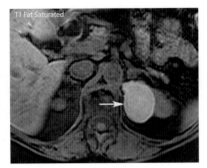

Figure 10.5   **Figure 10.6**

Findings

▸ A well-defined homogeneous left upper renal lesion (arrow in Figures 10.5 and 10.6) is noted; it is hyperintense on T2-weighted (Figure 10.1), nonfat-suppressed (Figure 10.2), and fat-suppressed T1-weighted (Figure 10.3) images. The subtraction image obtained after contrast administration does not demonstrate any enhancement (Figure 10.4).

Differential Diagnosis

▸ Homogeneous high T2 signal intensity noted in the sharply delineated right renal lesion is characteristic of a cyst. However, simple cysts are hypointense on T1 imaging, and the lesion noted here is homogeneously hyperintense on fat-suppressed and nonfat-suppressed T1-weighted images. The T1 hyperintensity suggests the cyst contains hemorrhagic material. The contrast-enhanced subtraction image allows assessment of the cyst for enhancement by subtracting out the background high T1 signal. Lack of any enhancing component on the subtracted image indicates the benign nature of this hemorrhagic renal cyst.

Teaching Points

▸ T1 hyperintensity in a renal cyst indicates hemorrhagic or proteinaceous contents.
▸ On CT imaging, cysts with hemorrhagic or proteinaceous contents are hyperdense with attenuation >20 HU on unenhanced studies.
▸ Nonenhancing hemorrhagic renal cysts <3 cm are considered benign Bosniak II cysts.
▸ Nonenhancing hemorrhagic cysts that are completely intrarenal (as the wall cannot be appreciated) and those >3 cm are considered Bosniak IIF cysts. Bosniak IIF cysts have high likelihood of being benign but need to be followed to exclude malignancy.

Management

▸ Follow-up is needed only for Bosniak IIF cysts to exclude malignancy.

Further Reading
Israel GM, Bosniak MA. How I do it: evaluating renal masses. *Radiology*. 2005;236(2):441–450.

History

▶ 45-year-old man with family history of renal cancer

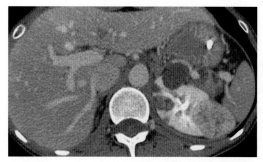

Figure 11.1

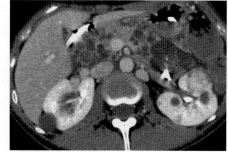

Figure 11.2

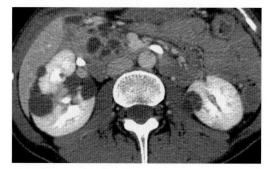

Figure 11.3

Case 11 Von Hippel–Lindau Syndrome

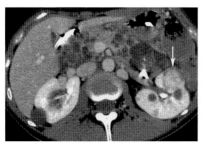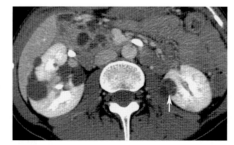

Figure 11.4   **Figure 11.5**

Findings

▶ Contrast-enhanced CT images (Figures 11.1, 11.2, and 11.3) show bilateral renal lesions, including simple and complex cysts and solid enhancing masses. Numerous pancreatic cysts are also present. Arrows point to a solid enhancing left renal neoplasm in Figure 11.4 and a complex cyst with enhancing septa in Figure 11.5.

Differential Diagnosis

▶ Combination of bilateral simple and complex renal cysts, solid renal lesions, and innumerable pancreatic cysts is characteristic of von Hippel–Lindau syndrome (VHL).

Teaching Points

▶ VHL is an autosomal dominant inherited multisystem disorder with an approximate incidence of 1 in 36000.

▶ VHL is characterized by development of various benign and malignant neoplasms, including central nervous system and retinal hemangioblastomas, endolymphatic sac tumors, renal cysts and tumors, pancreatic cysts and tumors, pheochromocytomas, and epididymal cystadenomas.

▶ Renal lesions are bilateral in 75% of patients with VHL. They include cysts, cystic renal cell carcinomas, and solid renal cell carcinomas (RCCs). RCC is seen in 35%–75% of patients with VHL. RCC is detected at a younger age (average age 35 years) compared with sporadic cases, which typically occur in the sixth decade.

▶ Foci of malignant cells are often present in benign-appearing renal cysts. All cysts in VHL are potentially premalignant.

▶ RCC and complications of cerebellar hemangioblastomas are the most common causes of mortality in VHL.

▶ Pancreatic lesions in VHL include cysts, serous cystadenomas, neuroendocrine tumors, and, rarely, adenocarcinoma. Incidence varies from 0% to 77% in different families.

▶ Pheochromocytomas in VHL patients are often multiple and may be ectopic.

Management

▶ Due to multiplicity of lesions, RCC in VHL is treated with nephron-sparing surgery or ablative procedures. One algorithm suggests resection of all lesions in a kidney once a lesion reaches a 3-cm size threshold.

Further Reading

Leung RS, Biswas SV, Duncan M, Rankin S. Imaging features of von Hippel–Lindau disease. *Radiographics*. 2008;28(1):65–79.

History

▶ 45-year-old man with family history of progressive renal dysfunction

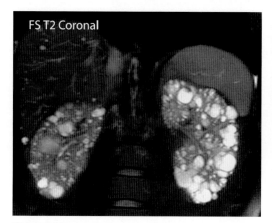

Figure 12.1

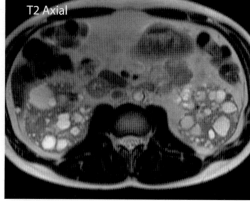

Figure 12.2

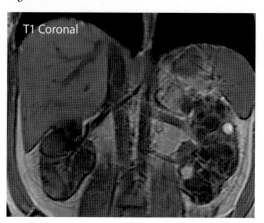

Figure 12.3

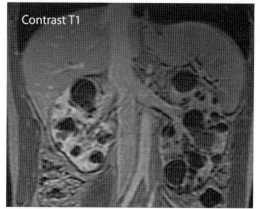

Figure 12.4

Case 12   Autosomal Dominant Polycystic Kidney Disease

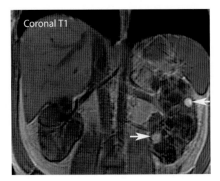

Coronal T1

Figure 12.5

Findings

▶ Fat-suppressed T2-weighted (Figure 12.1), nonfat-suppressed T2-weighted (Figure 12.2), T1-weighted (Figure 12.3), and post-contrast T1-weighted (Figure 12.4) images show bilateral enlarged kidneys replaced by innumerable cysts. Most cysts are simple (T2 hyperintense, T1 hypointense). A few T1 hyperintense hemorrhagic cysts are present (arrows in Figure 12.5). Small hepatic cysts are seen (Figure 12.1).

Differential Diagnosis

▶ Acquired cystic renal disease has multiple small cysts in atrophic kidneys and occurs in patients with renal failure. Multiorgan involvement with hepatic cysts in addition to large bilateral renal cysts, as seen in this patient, is typical of autosomal dominant polycystic kidney disease (ADPKD).

Teaching Points

▶ ADPKD is a dominantly inherited systemic disease with an incidence of 1:700 to 1:1000. Each offspring has a 50% chance of inheriting this disease.
▶ It is characterized by multiple epithelial-lined renal cysts, resulting in gradual massive kidney enlargement; this leads to kidney failure in the majority of individuals by the fifth or sixth decade.
▶ ADPKD is caused by mutation in the PKD1 gene in 85% of patients and in the PKD2 gene in 15% of patients. ADPKD2 has a less severe course of disease with a later mean age of diagnosis.
▶ Extra renal cysts are most often found in the liver, spleen, pancreas, and thyroid. Intracranial aneurysms are present in 5%–7% of patients.
▶ Ultrasound criteria for ADPKD1 in patients at risk are at least two cysts in one kidney or one cyst in each kidney at age <30 years, or at least two cysts in each kidney at age 30–59 years, or at least four cysts in each kidney at age >59 years.
▶ Fewer than two renal cysts exclude ADPKD in "at risk" patients aged >40 years.
▶ Imaging studies estimate renal volume, which is predictive of subsequent rate of progression and risk of renal insufficiency.
▶ ADPKD patients are not at higher risk of malignancy.

Management

▶ No treatment has yet been shown to slow disease progression, but much work is in progress.

Further Reading
Chapman AB, Wei W. Imaging approaches to patients with polycystic kidney disease. *Semin Nephrol.* 2011;31(3):237–244.

History

▶ 56-year-old man post-radiofrequency ablation of left renal cell carcinoma; 1 month (Figures 13.1–13.3) and 6 months (Figures 13.4–13.6) post-ablation MR images are provided

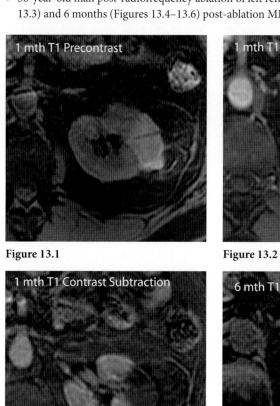

1 mth T1 Precontrast

Figure 13.1

1 mth T1 Contrast

Figure 13.2

1 mth T1 Contrast Subtraction

Figure 13.3

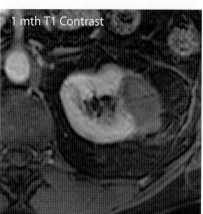

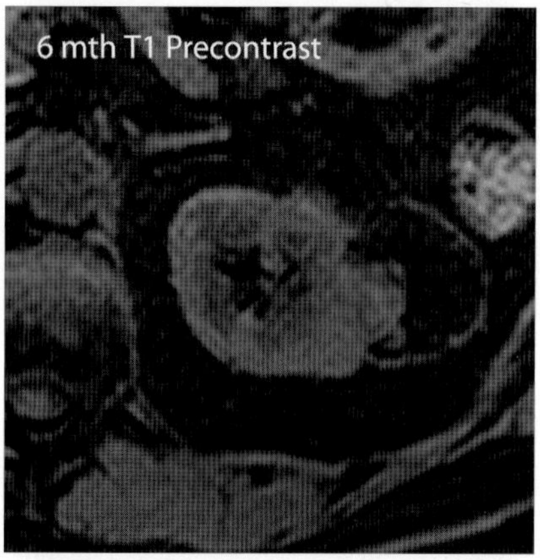

6 mth T1 Precontrast

Figure 13.4

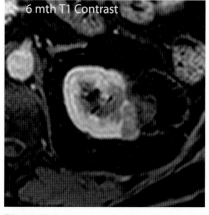

6 mth T1 Contrast

Figure 13.5

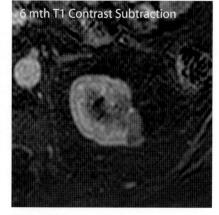

6 mth T1 Contrast Subtraction

Figure 13.6

Case 13 Post-Ablation Renal Cell Carcinoma Recurrence

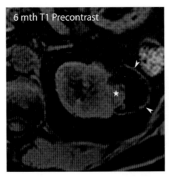

Figure 13.7

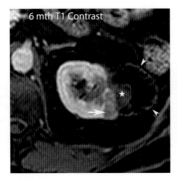

Figure 13.8

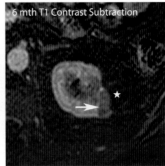

Figure 13.9

Findings

► One-month post-ablation–unenhanced T1-weighted image (Figure 13.1) shows T1 high signal within the ablation zone. On contrast-enhanced image (Figure 13.2), the high signal in the ablation zone persists. Corresponding subtraction image (Figure 13.3) does not show any enhancement in the ablation zone.

► Six-month post-ablation–unenhanced T1-weighted image (Figures 13.4 and 13.7) shows peripheral rim demarcating the ablation zone (arrowheads). Nodular high signal is seen in the medial aspect of the ablation zone (asterisk). Contrast-enhanced image (Figures 13.5 and 13.8) redemonstrates the peripheral rim (arrowheads) and high signal nodule in the medial aspect (asterisk). Additional nodular hypoenhancing component is apparent along the posteromedial margin of the ablation zone (arrow). Corresponding subtraction image (Figures 13.6 and 13.9) shows no enhancement in the peripheral rim or medial nodular component. Persistent nodular enhancement is identified along the posteromedial margin (arrow).

Differential Diagnosis

► High T1 signal filling the ablation zone on the 1-month post-ablation MR image (Figure 13.1) completely subtracts out on the post-contrast subtraction image. This is consistent with hemorrhage or devitalized tissue, an expected sequela of ablation. There is no enhancement to suggest residual disease on the 1-month MR image.

► On the 6-month follow-up MR image, the high T1 nodular component in the medial aspect of the ablation zone (asterisk) may appear concerning for recurrent tumor on the noncontrast and post-contrast images. However, the subtraction image does not show enhancement, suggesting that it represents devitalized tissue/clot and not viable tumor. Nodular enhancement along the posteromedial margin zone (arrow) shows enhancement both on the post-contrast and subtraction images. This is consistent with tumor recurrence at the margin of the ablation zone.

Teaching Points

► Image-guided ablation of renal cell carcinoma is performed in patients with early-stage tumors who are poor surgical candidates, have marginal renal function, or are at risk of developing additional tumors.

► Ablation zones have a target appearance on follow-up scans with central nonenhancing T1 bright/T2 dark area surrounded by fat with a T1/T2 variable peripheral rim.

► Ablation zones involute with time.

Management

► Ablation or surgery

Further Reading

Wile GE, Leyendecker JR, Krehbiel KA, Dyer RB, Zagoria RJ. CT and MR imaging after imaging-guided thermal ablation of renal neoplasms. *Radiographics*. 2007;27(2):325–339.

History

► 35-year-old woman with flank pain

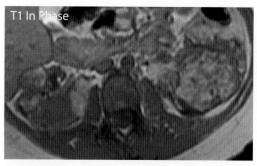

Figure 14.1

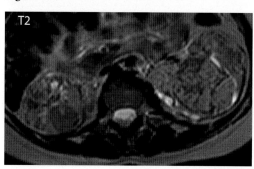

Figure 14.3

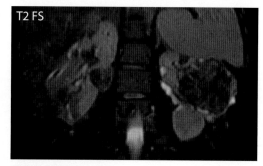

Figure 14.4

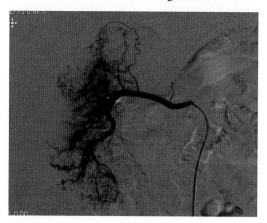

Figure 14.5

Case 14 Bilateral Renal Angiomyolipomas in Tuberous Sclerosis

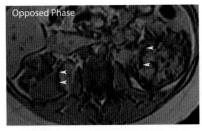

Figure 14.6

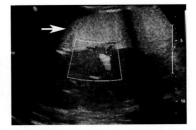

Figure 14.7

Findings

▶ MRI images show multiple bilateral renal lesions that are hyperintense on T1-weighted in-phase (Figure 14.1) and T2-weighted images (Figure 14.3). Lesions are etched in black at lesion–kidney interface on opposed-phase images (Figure 14.2; arrows in Figure 14.6) and hypointense on fat-suppressed T2-weighted images (Figure 14.4).

▶ Angiogram shows numerous tortuous tumor vessels and tumor blush throughout the right kidney (Figure 14.5).

▶ A Doppler ultrasound image from a different patient (Figure 14.7) shows a homogeneous, exophytic, echogenic lesion arising from the kidney. A large blood vessel is seen supplying the lesion.

Differential Diagnosis

▶ Findings are diagnostic of bilateral multiple fat-containing renal angiomyolipomas (AMLs), which are often seen in tuberous sclerosis.

Teaching Points

▶ AMLs are benign tumors of the kidney composed of varying amounts of fat, smooth muscle, and abnormal thick-walled blood vessels.

▶ AMLs are often multiple and bilateral in tuberous sclerosis patients; 55%–75% of tuberous sclerosis patients have renal AMLs.

▶ AMLs >4 cm are prone to bleeding.

▶ On opposed-phase MR imaging, the interface between macroscopic fat in AML and adjacent renal parenchyma is "etched in black." This is also known as India ink artifact and is due to the presence of fat and water protons within the same imaging voxel, resulting in signal loss at the interface. This is different from microscopic fat-containing lesions such as adrenal adenomas, which show conspicuous signal drop out of entire lesion on opposed-phase imaging.

▶ AMLs are hypointense on fat-suppressed MRI sequences.

▶ AMLs are usually homogeneously hyperechoic on ultrasound. This is not pathognomonic of AML since renal cell carcinoma can be hyperechoic.

▶ Approximately 95% of AMLs are hypervascular with tortuous, irregular, and aneurysmal vessels on angiography.

Management

▶ AMLs >4 cm commonly undergo renal-sparing surgery or renal arterial embolization, especially if there is evidence of hemorrhage or symptoms.

Further Reading
Prasad SR, Surabhi VR, Menias CO, Raut AA, Chintapalli KN. Benign renal neoplasms in adults: cross-sectional imaging findings. *AJR Am J Roentgenol.* 2008;190(1):158–164.

Case 15

History

- Asymptomatic 45-year-old female

Figure 15.1

Figure 15.2

Figure 15.3

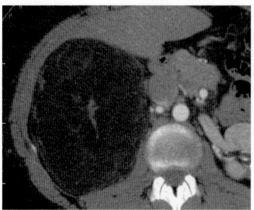

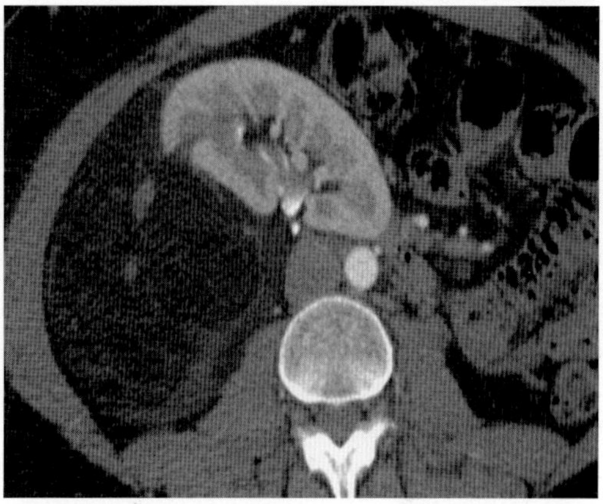

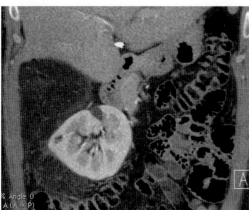

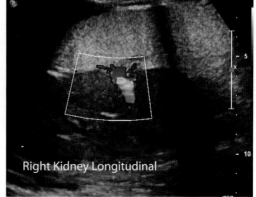

Figure 15.4

Case 15   Large Exophytic Renal Angiomyolipoma

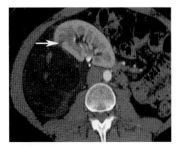
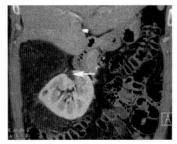
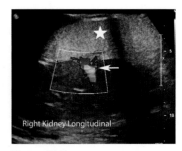

Figure 15.5   **Figure 15.6**   **Figure 15.7**

Findings

▶ Axial and coronal CT images (Figures 15.1–15.3) show a large, well-defined, predominantly fat-attenuation retroperitoneal mass containing small soft tissue–attenuation nodules. The mass displaces the right kidney anteriorly. A fatty wedge-shaped renal parenchymal defect is noted (arrow in Figures 15.5 and 15.6).

▶ Figure 15.4 is an ultrasound image from a different patient that shows a large homogeneously hyperechoic mass abutting the kidney (asterisk in Figure 15.7). Doppler flow is noted in a vascular pedicle (arrow in Figure 15.7) from the renal cortex into the mass.

Differential Diagnosis

▶ Differential diagnosis of a fat-containing retroperitoneal mass includes retroperitoneal liposarcoma and large exophytic renal angiomyolipoma (AML). Retroperitoneal liposarcomas can displace, compress, or distort the kidney but always have a smooth interface with the kidney. Demonstration of a wedge-shaped parenchyma defect confirms renal origin of the fatty lesion and establishes the diagnosis of renal AML in this patient.

▶ The homogeneously hyperechoic lesion noted in Figure 15.4 is a typical ultrasound feature of a fat-containing lesion. The presence of a tumoral vessel extending from the renal cortex into the fatty retroperitoneal favors the diagnosis of renal AML over retroperitoneal liposarcoma.

Teaching Points

▶ AMLs are benign renal tumors composed of varying amounts of fat, blood vessels, and smooth muscle.

▶ AMLs are more common in women.

▶ Eighty percent of AMLs are sporadic. Twenty percent are associated with tuberous sclerosis.

▶ Most AMLs are intraparenchymal, but 25% are exophytic. Large exophytic AMLs can mimic retroperitoneal liposarcomas.

▶ AMLs are prone to hemorrhage since they contain abnormal blood vessels.

Management

▶ Most AMLs are managed by observation alone. Large AMLs may be resected due to the risk of bleeding, which is higher in large tumors (>4 cm) and in the childbearing years. Embolization is also performed for acute hemorrhage.

Further Reading

Israel GM, Bosniak MA, Slywotzky CM, Rosen RJ. CT differentiation of large exophytic renal angiomyolipomas and perirenal liposarcomas. *AJR Am J Roentgenol.* 2002;179(3):769–773.

History

▶ 40-year-old female with abrupt onset of fever and flank pain (Figures 16.1–16.3); Figure 16.4 is from another patient with a different manifestation of the same disease

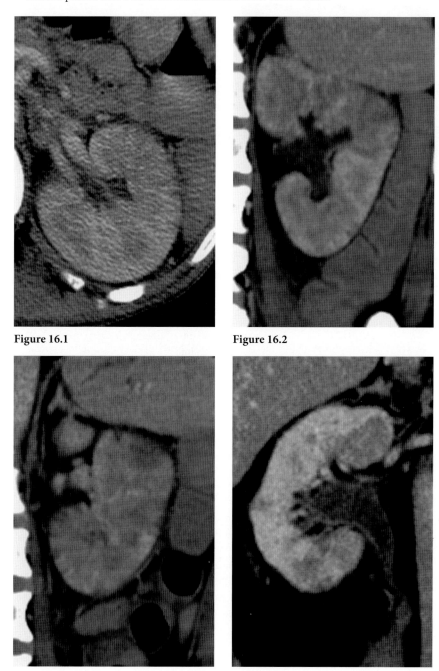

Figure 16.1

Figure 16.2

Figure 16.3

Figure 16.4

Case 16   Pyelonephritis

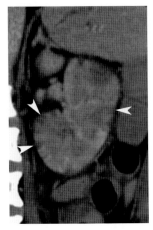

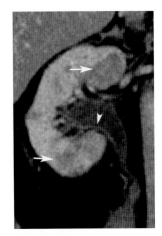

Figure 16.5   **Figure 16.6**

Findings

▶ Contrast-enhanced CT images (Figures 16.1–16.3) show an edematous, enlarged left kidney. A striated pattern of enhancement with multiple areas of streaky decreased enhancement that extend from the papilla to the cortex with adjacent normally enhancing parenchyma is seen (arrows in Figure 16.5).

▶ Figure 16.4 shows a different manifestation of the same disease. Multiple round hypoenhancing areas are present in the renal parenchyma (arrows in Figure 16.6). Diffuse urothelial enhancement is present (arrowhead in Figure 16.6).

Differential Diagnosis

▶ The differential diagnosis of striated nephrogram includes acute pyelonephritis, urinary obstruction, renal vein thrombosis, renal contusion, vasculitis, and hypotension. The clinical presentation confirms the diagnosis of acute pyelonephritis in this case. Acute pyelonephritis also presents as focal hypoenhancing areas. Diffuse urothelial enhancement suggests concomitant ureteropyelitis (both seen in Figure 16.5).

Teaching Points

▶ Acute pyelonephritis may be secondary to ascending (more common) or hematogeneous infection. Infection by gram-negative bacteria such as *Escherichia coli* suggest ascending infection, while gram-positive bacteria indicate hematogeneous spread.

▶ Typical presentation is abrupt onset of chills, fever, and flank pain with costovertebral tenderness, often in combination with dysuria.

▶ Imaging is not routinely required for the diagnosis and treatment of acute pyelonephritis.

▶ Imaging may be used to check for occult anatomic abnormalities and to assess severity and complications, especially in patients at risk for life-threatening complications.

▶ The pattern of alternate hypo- and hyperattenuating bands (striated nephrogram) seen in acute pyelonephritis reflects underlying interstitial nephritis. Inflammatory debris within the lumen, interstitial edema, and vasospasm cause tubular obstruction, which decreases flow of contrast and results in hypoenhancement in this region. On delayed imaging, a reversal may be noted and the original hypoenhancing areas may become hyperenhancing due to slow transit through these tubules.

Management

▶ Antibiotics

Further Reading
Craig WD, Wagner BJ, Travis MD. Pyelonephritis: radiologic–pathologic review. *Radiographics*. 2008;28(1):255–277.

History

▶ 46-year-old diabetic man with high-grade fever and flank pain

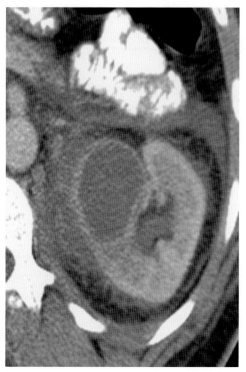

Figure 17.1

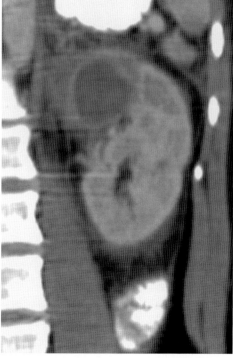

Figure 17.2

Case 17 Renal Abscess

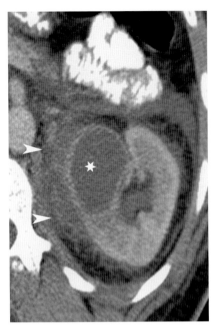

Figure 17.3

Findings

▶ Contrast-enhanced CT images (Figures 17.1 and 17.2) show a sharply marginated, unilocular, nonenhancing, low-attenuation lesion in the left renal parenchyma. Mild decreased enhancement is seen in the adjacent parenchyma. Prominent perinephric inflammatory fat stranding is present (arrowheads in Figure 17.3). Stranding and fluid are also noted along the perirenal fascia.

Differential Diagnosis

▶ Differential diagnosis for nonenhancing low-attenuation renal parenchymal lesion includes renal cyst and renal abscess. The prominent perinephric inflammation and clinical presentation are consistent with infection and confirm the diagnosis of renal abscess. Sharp margins suggest a mature abscess. Early immature abscesses appear as irregular, poorly marginated nonenhancing areas. A zone of decreased enhancement often surrounds an abscess, indicating infected, but not necrosed, parenchyma. Neoplastic processes such as lymphoma and transitional cell carcinoma are hypoenhancing, not associated with inflammatory changes, and usually more infiltrative.

Teaching Points

▶ Untreated or inadequately treated pyelonephritis may result in tissue necrosis and liquefaction, forming renal abscesses. Small foci often coalesce to form a larger abscess.
▶ Diabetics, immunocompromised patients, and those with obstructed systems are at higher risk.
▶ Seventy-five percent of renal abscesses occur in diabetics.
▶ Fifteen to twenty percent of patients with renal abscesses have negative urine cultures.
▶ CT is the preferred modality for the diagnosis and follow-up of renal abscesses to accurately identify extent and perinephric involvement.

Management

▶ Antibiotics are the first line of treatment. Percutaneous drainage may be attempted if antibiotic therapy fails.

Further Reading

Browne RF, Zwirewich C, Torreggiani WC. Imaging of urinary tract infection in the adult. *Eur Radiol.* 2004;14 (suppl 3):E168–183.

History

▶ 43-year-old man status post-renal transplant with fever

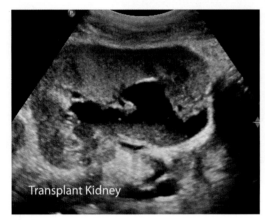

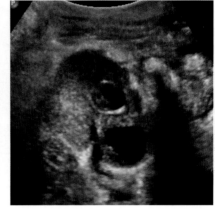

Figure 18.1

Figure 18.2

Case 18 Pyonephrosis

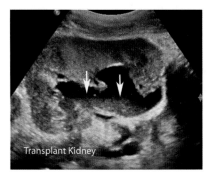

Figure 18.3

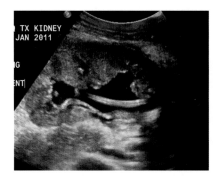

Figure 18.4

Findings

▸ Longitudinal and transverse ultrasound images of transplant kidney (Figures 18.1 and 18.2) show severe hydroureteronephrosis with layering of echogenic debris within the collecting system (arrows in Figure 18.3).

▸ Figure 18.4 is an ultrasound image obtained after retrograde decompression with ureteric stent. It shows clearing of the echogenic debris and reduction in hydronephrosis. Patient had obstruction at the ureteric anastomosis.

Differential Diagnosis

▸ In an immunocompromised patient with fever, echogenic layering debris within a dilated collecting system is likely to be diagnostic of pyonephrosis. Hemorrhage within the collecting system can have this ultrasound appearance but would present with hematuria.

Teaching Points

▸ Pyonephrosis describes an infected and obstructed renal collecting system.

▸ Ostruction can be due to stone, stricture, tumor, or surgical complication.

▸ Risk factors include immunosuppression and diabetes.

▸ Pyonephrosis presents with fever and flank pain, but 15% of patients are asymptomatic.

▸ The diagnosis should be suspected in any patient with known renal obstruction who develops fever and flank pain.

▸ Pyonephrosis can result in rapid and often permanent deterioration of renal function and can lead to septic shock.

▸ Presence of echogenic debris in the collecting system is the most reliable sign for pyonephrosis.

▸ Ultrasound has a sensitivity of 90% and specificity of 97% in the diagnosis of pyonephrosis versus simple hydronephrosis.

▸ CT imaging can show high-attenuation material within the collecting system, although it is difficult to differentiate between pyonephrosis and hydronephrosis based on attenuation values. Parenchymal and perinephric inflammatory changes, if present, are helpful.

Management

▸ Pyonephrosis is a surgical emergency and requires immediate antegrade or retrograde decompression in addition to parenteral antibiotics.

Further Reading

Craig WD, Wagner BJ, Travis MD. Pyelonephritis: radiologic-pathologic review. *Radiographics*. 2008;28(1):255–277.

History

▶ 45-year-old man with chronic left flank pain

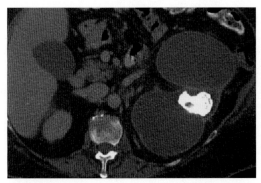

Figure 19.1

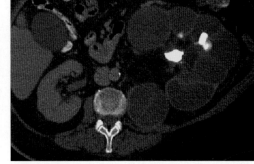

Figure 19.2

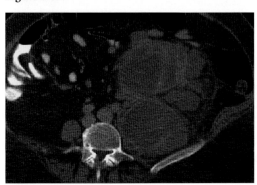

Figure 19.3

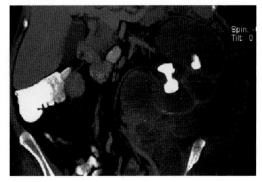

Figure 19.4

Case 19 Xanthogranulomatosis Pyelonephritis

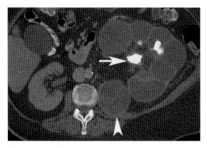 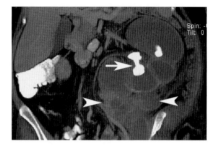

Figure 19.5   **Figure 19.6**

Findings

▶ Contrast-enhanced computed tomography images (Figures 19.1–19.4) show an enlarged left kidney with severe calyceal dilation with paper-thin parenchyma. Renal pelvis is contracted with a large obstructing staghorn calculus (arrows in Figures 19.5 and 19.6). Other large calyceal calculi are present. The left ureter is normal in caliber.

▶ Inflammation extends to the perinephric space and retroperitoneum with formation of retroperitoneal and psoas abscesses (Figure 19.3; arrowheads in Figures 19.5 and 19.6).

Differential Diagnosis

▶ The combination of a nonfunctioning enlarged kidney, central calculus within a contracted renal pelvis, expansion of the calyces, inflammatory changes in the perinephric fat, and psoas abscess is strongly suggestive of xanthogranulomatous pyelonephritis (XGP). Renal tuberculosis can cause dilated calyces, contracted pelvis, and psoas abscess but is associated with parenchymal and urothelial calcifications and not large obstructing pelvicalyceal calculi.

Teaching Points

▶ XGP is a form of chronic necrotizing granulomatous pyelonephritis caused by recurrent bacterial infection.

▶ No specific risk factors have been identified.

▶ Symptoms are nonspecific and include low-grade fever, malaise, flank pain, pyuria, and hematuria.

▶ XGP is characterized by the formation soft, yellow nodules that are composed of foamy lipid-laden macrophages.

▶ Most cases have renal pelvic calculus.

▶ Loss of renal function is due to global severe inflammation rather than obstruction. The dilated calyces are often filled with extensive inflammatory infiltrate rather than fluid.

▶ Atypical features include renal atrophy rather than enlargement, focal renal involvement, and absence of calculi.

▶ Extrarenal extension with psoas abscess and fistula to the skin or bowel are common complications.

Management

▶ Nephrectomy

Further Reading

Rajesh A, Jakanani G, Mayer N, Mulcahy K. Computed tomography findings in xanthogranulomatous pyelonephritis. *J Clin Imaging Sci.* 2011;1:45.

History

▶ 48-year-old diabetic woman status post-renal transplant with high-grade fever, flank pain, and confusion

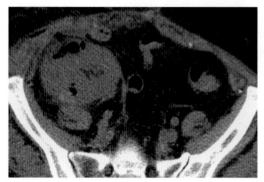

Figure 20.1

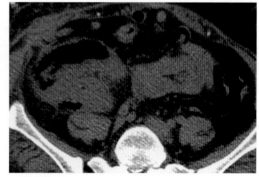

Figure 20.2

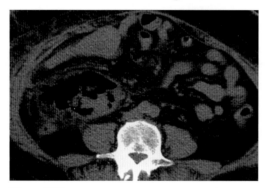

Figure 20.3

Case 20   Emphysematous Pyelonephritis

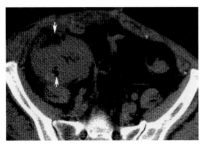

Figure 20.4

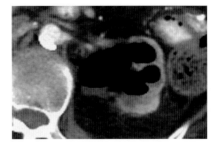

Figure 20.5

Findings

► Unenhanced CT images (Figures 20.1–20.3) show gas within the transplant renal parenchyma (arrows in Figure 20.4). There is extension of the predominantly gas-containing abscess into the perirenal tissues (Figure 20.3).

► Figure 20.5 shows a different patient with gas limited to the collecting system (emphysematous pyelitis).

Differential Diagnosis

► Differential diagnosis of gas within the kidney depends on location of the gas. Gas limited to the collecting system can be due to infection (emphysematous pyelitis; Figure 20.5), recent instrumentation, or fistula to the bowel. In this patient, gas is present within the renal parenchyma with extension into the perinephric space. This is characteristic of emphysematous pyelonephritis.

Teaching Points

► Emphysematous pyelonephritis is an acute, fulminant, necrotizing infection of the renal parenchyma and perirenal tissues.

► Eighty to ninety-six percent of patients with emphysematous pyelonephritis are diabetics. Immunosuppression due to any cause and obstruction are additional risk factors.

► *Escherichia coli* is the most common infecting organism.

► Emphysematous pyelonephritis can rapidly progress to sepsis and death. Overall mortality of emphysematous pyelonephritis is 25% (11%–42%).

► Infection-causing gas limited to the collecting system is known as emphysematous pyelitis. It has a much better prognosis compared with gas within the renal parenchyma (emphysematous pyelonephritis).

► Extension of gas or gas-containing abscess beyond the kidney has a worse prognosis than when gas is limited to the renal parenchyma.

► CT is the most specific and sensitive modality to detect the presence, location, and extent of gas.

Management

► Treatment of emphysematous pyelonephritis includes intravenous antibiotics, abscess drainage, and decompression of urinary tract obstruction. Nephrectomy is sometimes performed in patients at high risk and upon failure of conservative management.

Further Reading

Akhtar AL, Elsayes KM, Woodward S. AJR teaching file: diabetic patient presenting with right flank pain and fever. *AJR Am J Roentgenol*. 2010;194(6 suppl):WS31–33.

History

▶ 40-year-old human immunodeficiency virus (HIV)–infected man with rapidly deteriorating renal function

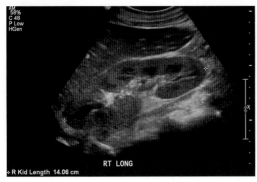

Figure 21.1

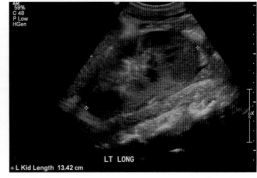

Figure 21.2

Case 21 Human Immunodeficiency Virus Associated Nephropathy

Findings

▶ Ultrasound images (Figures 21.1 and 21.2) show bilateral enlarged kidneys. The cortical echogenicity is increased and is greater than the adjacent liver.

Differential Diagnosis

▶ Differential diagnosis for bilateral large kidneys includes diabetes, acute glomerulonephritis, vasculitis, lymphoma, and HIV-associated nephropathy (HIVAN). In the HIV-infected population, increased renal echogenicity and size are indicators of HIVAN. Lymphoma is usually hypoechoic on ultrasound and most commonly forms focal masses. It also obliterates the renal architecture. Other diseases mentioned above are less common causes of renal dysfunction in HIV patients than HIVAN. These diseases also cause less increase in renal echotexture compared with HIVAN. Overall, the ultrasound findings favor HIVAN in this clinical setting, but the diagnosis should be confirmed by biopsy.

Teaching Points

▶ HIVAN is a disease with distinct pathological and imaging features seen in patients with HIV infection.
▶ It is the leading cause of renal failure in HIV-positive patients and accounts for 40% of HIV-related renal disease.
▶ Other causes of renal impairment in HIV patients include infections, drug side effects, malignancy, and renal conditions that affect general population.
▶ HIVAN has a very strong predilection for the African American population.
▶ It is more common in patients with a CD4 count <200 but can occur in early stages of infection.
▶ HIVAN results in very rapid deterioration of renal function.
▶ Increased renal echogenicity on ultrasound is a typical feature of HIVAN. Normal renal echotexture almost excludes the disease, while severely increased echogenicity has high specificity.
▶ Large renal size is a feature of HIVAN.

Management

▶ Highly active antiretroviral therapy

Further Reading
Symeonidou C, Standish R, Sahdev A, Katz RD, Morlese J, Malhotra A. Imaging and histopathologic features of HIV-related renal disease. *Radiographics*. 2008;28(5):1339–1354.

History

▶ 25-year-old woman with nasal bleeding, hematuria, and positive cytoplasmic antineutrophil cytoplasmic antibody (c-ANCA) titer; CT imaging was followed by MRI after a 1-month interval

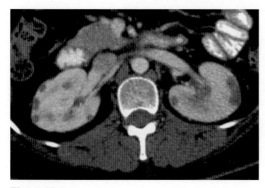

Figure 22.1

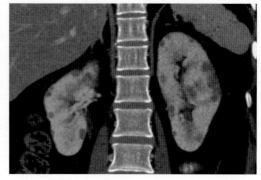

Figure 22.2

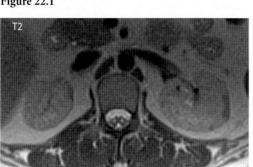

Figure 22.3

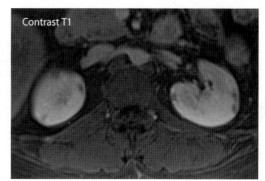

Figure 22.4

Case 22 Wegener's Granulomatosis

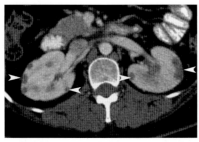

Figure 22.5

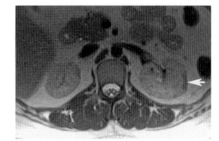

Figure 22.6

Findings

▶ Contrast-enhanced CT images (Figures 22.1 and 22.2) show multiple, bilateral, hypoenhancing, endophytic, renal cortical lesions (arrow in Figure 22.5).

▶ T2-weighted (Figure 22.3) and T1 fat-suppressed–enhanced (Figure 22.4) images from MRI performed 1 month later show interval decrease in the size of the lesions. The lesions are heterogeneously hypointense on T2-weighted imaging (arrow in Figure 22.6).

Differential Diagnosis

▶ Differential diagnosis for multiple, bilateral, hypoenhancing, renal cortical lesions includes hypovascular renal neoplasms such as lymphoma, multifocal papillary renal cell carcinoma and metastases, infection, and inflammatory diseases, including sarcoidosis and Wegener's granulomatosis. Although the imaging features are nonspecific, the decrease in number and size of renal lesions on the follow-up MRI suggests a nonneoplastic etiology. In this patient, the clinical presentation is characteristic of Wegener's granulomatosis, and the renal lesions are compatible with confluent necrotizing granulomas seen in this disease.

Teaching Points

▶ Wegener's granulomatosis is a systemic disease characterized by necrotizing granulomatous inflammation of the upper and lower respiratory tracts and vasculitis of small and medium-sized vessels.

▶ c-ANCA is positive in 85%–90% of patients.

▶ Renal involvement is seen in 80% and lung involvement in 90% of patients with Wegener's granulomatosis.

▶ Clinical manifestations of renal involvement include hematuria, proteinuria, and acute renal failure.

▶ Renal involvement usually manifests as focal segmental glomerulonephritis.

▶ Most patients with renal involvement do not have findings on imaging.

▶ Necrotizing renal granulomas (as seen in this case) are an uncommon manifestation of renal involvement in Wegener's granulomatosis. These appear as focal hypoenhancing renal lesions on imaging.

Management

▶ Immunosuppression

Further Reading

Fairbanks KD, Hellmann DB, Fishman EK, Ali SZ, Stone JH. Wegener's granulomatosis presenting as a renal mass. *AJR Am J Roentgenol.* 2000;174(6):1597–1598.

History

▶ 20-year-old male with intermittent hematuria, flank pain, and low-grade fever

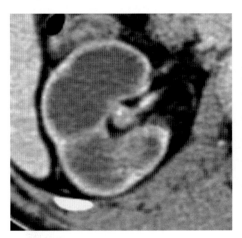

Figure 23.1

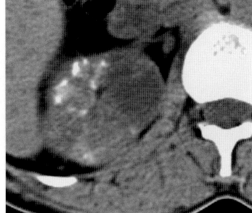

Figure 23.2

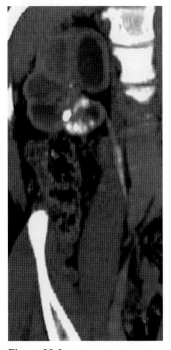

Figure 23.3

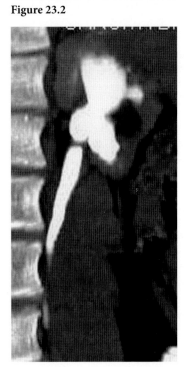

Figure 23.4

Case 23 Renal Tuberculosis

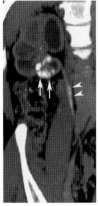 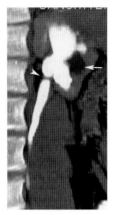

Figure 23.5   **Figure 23.6**

Findings

▶ CT urogram images (Figures 23.1–23.3) reveal severe right renal caliectasis with thin rim of residual parenchyma. No excretion of contrast is seen. Parenchymal calcification with lobar distribution is present (arrows in Figure 23.5). The renal pelvis is contracted with calcific foci. The right ureter is thickened and rigid with partially calcified walls.

▶ Excretory-phase CT image in a different patient shows ureteropelvic junction (UPJ) stricture (Figure 23.4, arrowhead in Figure 23.6) with proximal hydronephrosis. A dilated unopacified calyx is present (phantom calyx, arrows in Figure 23.6), likely due to infundibular stenosis.

Differential Diagnosis

▶ Differential diagnosis of a nonfunctioning kidney with caliectasis and contracted renal pelvis includes chronic infectious processes such as xanthogranulomatous pyelonephritis and tuberculosis. Presence of renal parenchymal calcification (particularly in lobar distribution) and thick, calcified ureter (pipe-stem ureter) favor diagnosis of genitourinary tuberculosis. Multifocal strictures (infundibular, UPJ, and ureteral) are characteristic of tuberculosis. Staghorn calculus is present in most cases of xanthogranulomatous pyelonephritis.

Teaching Points

▶ Genitourinary tuberculosis accounts for 15%–20% of cases of tuberculosis outside the lungs; 25% of patients with genitourinary tuberculosis have history of pulmonary infection.

▶ A long latent period (5–40 years) is often present between infection and expression of genitourinary disease. Dysuria, hematuria, and pyuria are common presentations.

▶ Renal infection is secondary to seeding from the bloodstream. Tiny tuberculomas may heal or they may enlarge and rupture into nephrons, causing bacilluria. Calyceal irregularity and papillary necrosis are the earliest imaging manifestations. Infection of the walls of the calyces, pelvis, and ureter causes mucosal inflammation with ulceration, granuloma formation, and finally fibrosis with stricture. Granulomas may form caseous or calcified parenchymal masses.

▶ End-stage renal tuberculosis results in a nonfunctioning hydronephrotic kidney or small, calcified kidney (putty kidney).

▶ Bladder involvement causes small-capacity irregular bladder (thimble bladder).

Management

▶ Multidrug antituberculous treatment; the role of nephrectomy is controversial

Further Reading
Gibson MS, Puckett ML, Shelly ME. Renal tuberculosis. *Radiographics*. 2004;24(1):251–256.

Case 24

History

- 38-year-old male, native of the Middle East, presents with right flank pain

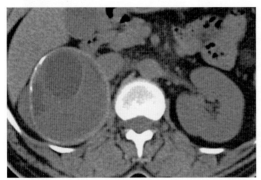

Figure 24.1

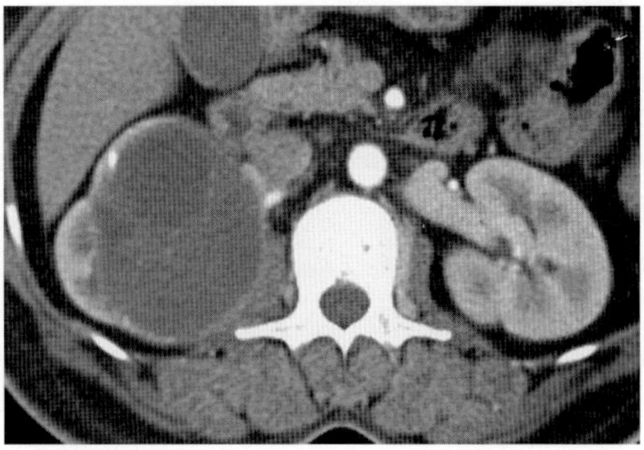

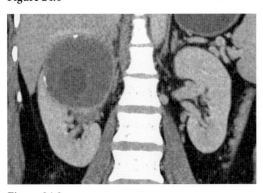

Figure 24.2

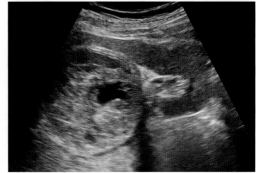

Figure 24.3

Figure 24.4

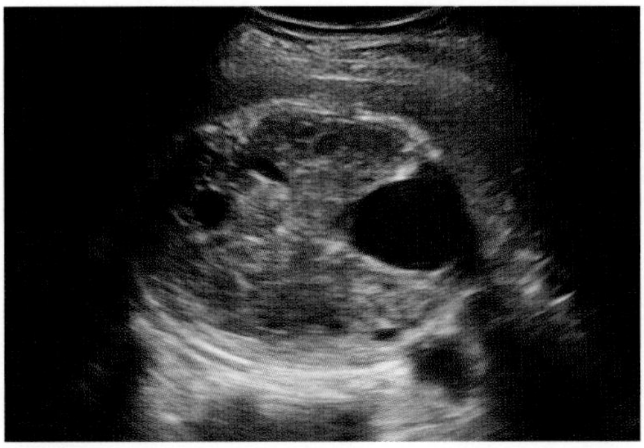

Figure 24.5

Case 24 Renal Hydatid Disease

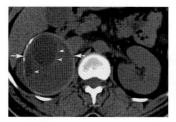

Figure 24.6

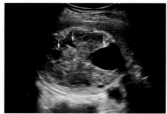

Figure 24.7

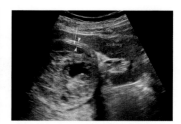

Figure 24.8

Findings

▶ Unenhanced and enhanced CT images (Figures 24.1–24.3) show a well-defined, partially exophytic right renal cyst with mildly thick hyperdense walls (best appreciated on unenhanced image) and curvilinear wall calcification (arrows in Figure 24.6). Small, well-demarcated, low-attenuation round locules/cysts are present within the large cyst (arrowheads in Figure 24.6).

▶ Longitudinal and oblique (Figures 24.4 and 24.5) ultrasound images reveal a predominant echogenic component/matrix with small anechoic locules/cysts (arrows in Figure 24.7). The wall shows double echogenic lines with hypoechoic layer in between (Figure 24.8).

Differential Diagnosis

▶ Differential diagnosis of multiloculated cyst includes neoplastic Bosniak III cyst, renal abscess, and renal hydatid cyst. Renal abscesses have a different presentation and do not have such well-demarcated walls and septa. Presence of low-attenuation round daughter cysts within the mother cyst, hyperdense cyst wall, and ring-like wall calcification in a native of an endemic region suggest diagnosis of hydatid disease over a neoplastic cyst. Double-layer wall and echogenic matrix (hydatid matrix) with scattered daughter cysts seen on ultrasound are features of hydatid disease.

Teaching Points

▶ Hydatid disease is caused primarily by the larval stage of *Echinococcus granulosus* and is endemic in the Mediterranean, Middle East, India, Africa, and Australia.

▶ Hydatid disease commonly affects the liver (75%), but kidneys are affected in 3% of patients.

▶ Cyst wall consists of outer pericyst formed by host inflammation and inner endocyst. The germinal layer of the endocyst forms daughter cysts that contain protoscolices.

▶ Hydatid cysts may be unilocular (type 1), multilocular with lower attenuation daughter cysts (type 2), or completely calcified (type 3, dead parasite).

▶ Hydatid matrix separates daughter cysts and contains detached membranes, hydatid sand, and scolices. Matrix is mixed echogenic and, when predominant, may mimic a solid mass. Identification of daughter cysts or membranes helps to establish the diagnosis.

▶ Cyst rupture can cause disease dissemination and/or anaphylaxis.

Management

▶ Surgical excision

Further Reading

Pedrosa I, Saíz A, Arrazola J, Ferreirós J, Pedrosa CS. Hydatid disease: radiologic and pathologic features and complications. *RadioGraphics.* 2000;20(3):795–817.

History

▸ 40-year-old man with history of hyperparathyroidism

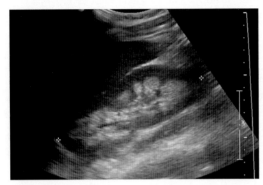

Figure 25.1

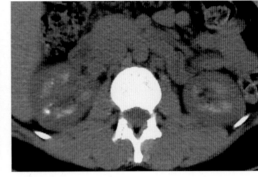

Figure 25.2

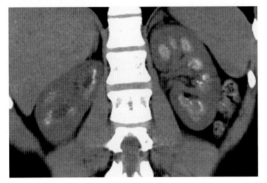

Figure 25.3

Case 25 Medullary Nephrocalcinosis

Findings

► Ultrasound image of the right kidney (Figure 25.1) shows increased echogenicity of the renal medulla.
► Unenhanced CT images (Figures 25.2 and 25.3) reveal calcium deposition in the renal pyramids bilaterally.

Differential Diagnosis

► Hyperechoic renal medulla on ultrasound has been described in medullary nephrocalcinosis and gout. Identification of bilateral medullary calcifications on CT confirms the diagnosis of medullary nephrocalcinosis in this patient. Medullary nephrocalcinosis should be differentiated from cortical nephrocalcinosis. Cortical nephrocalcinosis is much less common and is characterized by renal cortical calcifications with sparing of the medulla.

Teaching Points

► Medullary nephrocalcinosis is caused by calcium deposition in the renal pyramids.
► Any cause of hypercalcemia and/or hypercalcuria predisposes to calcium deposition in the medulla. Hyperparathyroidism and type 1 renal tubular acidosis are common causes of medullary nephrocalcinosis. Hypervitaminosis D, sarcoidosis, and milk alkali syndrome are rare causes.
► Medullary sponge kidney is another common cause of medullary nephrocalcinosis. Stasis in ectatic renal tubules found in this disease results in calcium deposition, leading to medullary nephrocalcinosis. Underlying metabolic abnormality is not present in these patients.
► Medullary nephrocalcinosis is often asymptomatic. Symptoms are related to underlying etiology.
► Calcium deposits can rupture into the calyceal system and become urinary tract calculi. These patients often present with renal colic.

Management

► Management of underlying metabolic abnormality

Further Reading
Toyoda K, Miyamoto Y, Ida M, Tada S, Utsunomiya M. Hyperechoic medulla of the kidneys. *Radiology*. 1989;173:431–434.

History

- 50-year-old male with chronic renal failure

Right Kidney Longitudinal

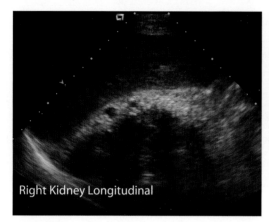

Figure 26.1

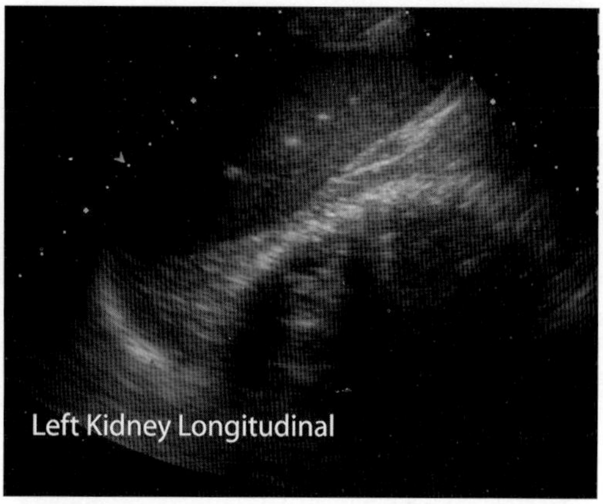

Left Kidney Longitudinal

Figure 26.2

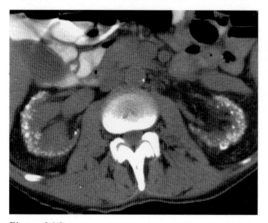

Figure 26.3

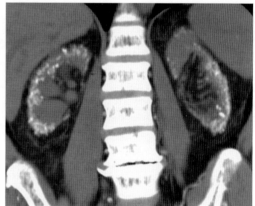

Figure 26.4

Case 26   Cortical Nephrocalcinosis

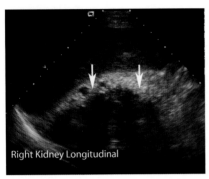

Right Kidney Longitudinal

Figure 26.5

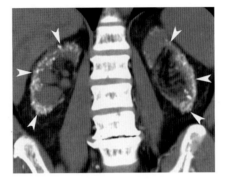

Figure 26.6

Findings

▶ Grayscale ultrasound images of kidneys (Figures 26.1 and 26.2) show increased cortical echogenicity with dense post-acoustic shadowing (arrows in Figure 26.5).

▶ Axial and coronal unenhanced CT images (Figures 26.3 and 26.4) show bilateral atrophic kidneys with extensive renal parenchymal calcifications predominantly involving the renal cortex (arrowheads in Figure 26.6).

Differential Diagnosis

▶ Renal calcification can be within the collecting system when it represents nephrolithiasis or within the renal parenchyma when it represents nephrocalcinosis. Parenchymal calcification can be within renal medulla (medullary nephrocalcinosis) or cortex (cortical nephrocalcinosis). In this patient, the parenchymal calcifications primarily involve the renal cortex, which is consistent with cortical nephrocalcinosis. The underlying cause was chronic glomerulonephritis.

Teaching Points

▶ Chronic glomerulonephritis, acute cortical necrosis (due to ischemia, sepsis, toxins), renal allograft rejection, and oxalosis are the most common causes of cortical nephrocalcinosis.

▶ Ultrasound demonstrates increased cortical echogenicity, with advanced cases showing post-acoustic shadowing.

▶ CT patterns of cortical nephrocalcinosis include a thin peripheral cortical band of calcification, thin rims of calcification along inner and outer margin of cortex (tramline tracks), or punctate random cortical calcifications.

▶ Calcifications appear as signal voids on MRI and may be difficult to identify.

Management

▶ Management of underlying condition

Further Reading

Schepens D, Verswijvel G, Kuypers D, Vanrenterghem Y. Images in nephrology. Renal cortical nephrocalcinosis. *Nephrol Dial Transplant*. 2000;15(7):1080–1082.

History

▶ 50-year-old diabetic man with microhematuria

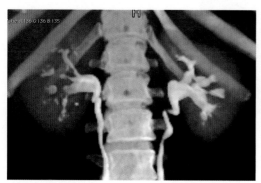

Figure 27.1

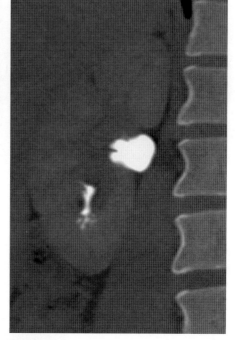

Figure 27.2

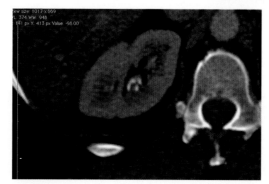

Figure 27.3

Case 27   Renal Papillary Necrosis

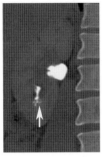 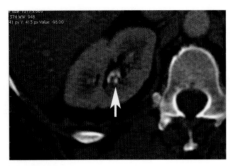

Figure 27.4   **Figure 27.5**

Findings

▶ Volume-rendered reconstruction coronal image of the excretory phase of a CT urogram (Figure 27.1) shows bilateral irregular calyces with contrast-filled clefts. Coronal reformatted and axial CT images (Figures 27.2 and 27.3) show contrast from the collecting system extending to small cavities in the papillae (arrows in Figures 27.4 and 27.5).

Differential Diagnosis

▶ Differential diagnosis of bilateral, multiple, calyceal irregularities includes papillary necrosis and medullary sponge kidney. Medullary sponge kidney is an asymptomatic developmental condition that results in ectasia of renal tubules. This gives a "paintbrush" appearance of the medulla on the excretory phase. Advanced disease rarely results in cystic dilation of tubules, which is difficult to differentiate from papillary necrosis. Multiple, bilateral contrast-filled clefts extending into medulla, as seen in this patient, is characteristic of papillary necrosis. The clinical profile of diabetes with microhematuria also fits papillary necrosis. Calyceal diverticula are smooth cystic cavities that communicate with the collecting system. They are not usually multiple and do not cause calyceal irregularity.

Teaching Points

▶ Papillary necrosis results from ischemia due to decreased blood flow to renal pyramids.
▶ Causes include diabetes, analgesic abuse, sickle cell disease, pyelonephritis, renal vein thrombosis, tuberculosis, and obstructive uropathy.
▶ Detection requires opacification of the collecting system with contrast. In the past, this was done by intravenous urogram; today it is obtained by excretory-phase imaging during CT urography.
▶ Early ischemic change in the medulla is reversible if underlying metabolic or infectious cause of ischemia is treated.
▶ As the disease advances, clefts form from the fornices to the papillae. Eventually, papillae slough into the collecting system and appear as filling defects on imaging.
▶ Papillae are nidus for calcification and may be passed as small stones.
▶ Papillary necrosis heals by scarring and results in blunt-tipped calices and cortical thinning.

Management

▶ Management of underlying condition to prevent renal scarring and parenchymal loss

Further Reading

Jung DC, Kim SH, Jung SI, Hwang SI, Kim SH. Renal papillary necrosis: review and comparison of findings at multi-detector row CT and intravenous urography. *Radiographics*. 2006;26(6):1827–1836.

History

► 29-year-old woman with an incidental renal lesion

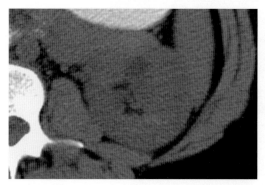

Figure 28.1

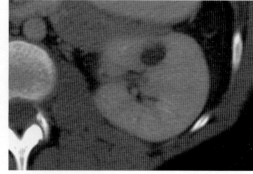

Figure 28.2

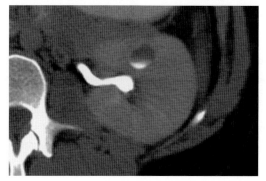

Figure 28.3

Case 28   Calyceal Diverticulum

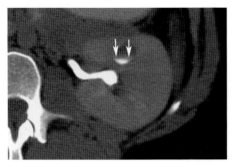

Figure 28.4

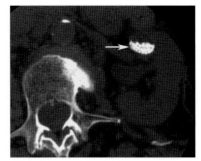

Figure 28.5

Findings

▶ Unenhanced (Figure 28.1) and nephrographic-phase (Figure 28.2) CT images show a well-defined, round, low-attenuation, nonenhancing, simple-appearing renal cystic lesion. Excretory-phase image (Figure 28.3) shows layering of excreted contrast within the cystic structure (arrows in Figure 28.4).

▶ Figure 28.5 is from a different patient. Multiple calculi are noted within a cystic renal lesion (arrow).

Differential Diagnosis

▶ Differential diagnosis of a low-attenuation, well-defined renal parenchymal lesion includes simple renal cyst and calyceal diverticulum. This lesion has the characteristics of a simple cyst on the unenhanced and nephrographic-phase scans. Layering of contrast within the cyst on the delayed phase indicates communication with the collecting system. This is pathognomonic of a calyceal diverticulum. Figure 28.5 shows layering of multiple calculi within a calyceal diverticulum in a different patient.

Teaching Points

▶ Calyceal diverticula are urine-containing cavities in the renal parenchyma that communicate with the collecting system.

▶ Etiology is unknown and likely represents a developmental anomaly.

▶ Incidence is 2 to 4 per 1000 intravenous urograms.

▶ Diverticula usually arise from the calyceal fornix but may arise from the infundulum or renal pelvis.

▶ Most calyceal diverticula are asymptomatic.

▶ Calyceal diverticula are prone to infection and calculi formation due to urinary stasis.

▶ Layering of milk of calcium may be seen within the diverticula.

▶ On ultrasound, calyceal diverticula have a cyst-like appearance. Presence of mobile echogenic foci within (milk of calcium or calculi) suggests the diagnosis.

▶ On CT, delayed excretory-phase imaging is essential to demonstrate communication with collecting system.

Management

▶ Symptomatic patients undergo surgery for removal of calculi and destruction of diverticula.

Further Reading

Stunell H, McNeill G, Browne RF, Grainger R, Torreggiani WC. The imaging appearances of calyceal diverticula complicated by uroliathasis. *Br J Radiol.* 2010;83(994):888–894.

History

▶ 45-year-old man following motorcycle accident

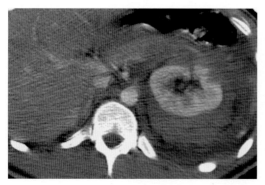

Figure 29.1

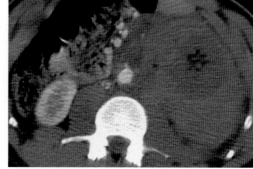

Figure 29.2

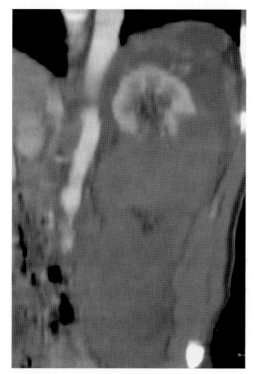

Figure 29.3

Case 29   Renal Trauma

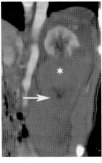 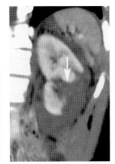

Figure 29.4   **Figure 29.5**

Findings

▸ Contrast-enhanced CT images (Figures 29.1–29.4) show a "shattered kidney" with complete transection and separation of renal parenchymal fragments. A large hematoma (asterisk in Figure 29.4) separates the enhancing upper kidney from devascularized lower kidney (arrow in Figure 29.4). A large perinephric hematoma is present.

▸ Figure 29.5 is from a different patient. A deep parenchymal laceration (arrow) extends to the collecting system. Perinephric hematoma is present.

Differential Diagnosis

▸ Large lacerations that transect the kidney with separation of the fragments and nonenhancement of a large portion of the kidney, as noted in this patient, can be considered a shattered kidney. Shattered kidney is grade 5 renal trauma. Grade 4 injury is less extensive and includes deep parenchymal lacerations with collecting system involvement, as seen in Figure 29.5.

Teaching Points

▸ The renal injury scale proposed by American Association for Surgery of Trauma (1989) is used to grade renal trauma.

▸ Grade 1 includes parenchymal contusions and nonexpanding subcapsular hematomas (approximately 82% of renal injuries).

▸ Grade 2 includes superficial cortical lacerations <1 cm deep and nonexpanding perirenal hematomas.

▸ Grade 3 includes lacerations >1 cm deep without extension into the collecting system or evidence of urinary extravasation.

▸ Grade 4 includes deep lacerations that involve the collecting system or main renal artery/vein injury with contained hemorrhage.

▸ Grade 5 includes shattered kidney and renal devascularization due to avulsion.

▸ Vascular injury is seen in 5.5% of renal trauma.

▸ Delayed excretory-phase CT is recommended when portal venous-phase CT reveals deep parenchymal laceration or large perinephric hematoma/collection. This identifies collecting system injury and urine leak, differentiating grade 3 from grade 4 trauma.

Management

▸ Even severe renal injuries are managed conservatively, unless there is intraperitoneal extension. Surgery is also performed for life-threatening renal hemorrhage, extensive (>50%) devascularized renal parenchyma, urine leak not controlled by conservative means, and arterial thrombosis.

Further Reading
Moore EE, Cogbill TH, Malangoni MA, et al. Organ injury scaling. *Surg Clin North Am.* 1995;75(2):293–303.

Case 30

History

► 55-year-old man with history of heart disease presents with right flank pain and hematuria

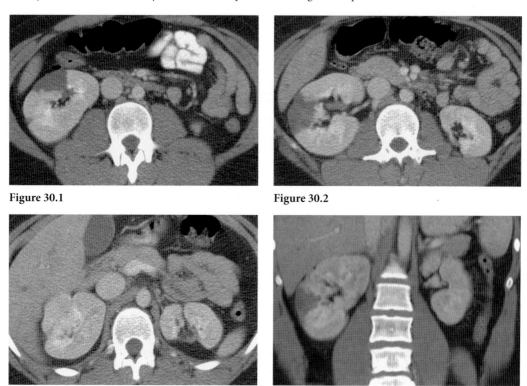

Figure 30.1

Figure 30.2

Figure 30.3

Figure 30.4

Case 30   Acute and Chronic Renal Infarcts

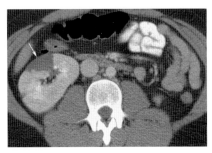 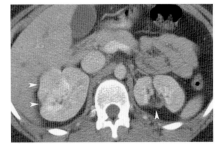

Figure 30.5   **Figure 30.6**

Findings

▶ Contrast-enhanced CT images (Figures 30.1–30.4) show well-demarcated, cortically based, wedge-shaped, peripheral, nonenhancing areas in the right kidney (arrow in Figure 30.5). Areas of focal parenchymal loss and scarring are present in both kidneys (arrowheads in Figure 30.6).

Differential Diagnosis

▶ Nonenhancing, wedge-shaped, cortically based areas in the kidney with areas of focal parenchymal loss and scarring are highly suggestive of acute segmental infarcts in a kidney with past vascular insults. Renal abscesses can have similar clinical presentation but do not have wedge-shaped configuration. Transitional cell carcinoma can present as hypoenhancing parenchymal lesions in patients with hematuria but are more centrally located without the wedge-shaped configuration.

Teaching Points

▶ Kidneys are vulnerable to developing infarcts due to the "end organ" nature of blood supply with extremely limited collaterals from extrarenal sites.
▶ The most common cause of renal infarction is thromboembolism from cardiovascular disease. Approximately 50% of patients with renal infarcts have atrial fibrillation. Infective endocarditis, complex aortic plaques, and left ventricular thrombi are other sources of thromboembolism.
▶ Acute renal infarction presents with flank pain, nausea, hematuria, leukocytosis, and elevated serum lactate dehydrogenase.
▶ Global renal infarcts involve more than 50% of the renal cortex.
▶ Cortical or subcapsular rim sign refers to a 2- to 4-mm ribbon of peripheral-enhancing cortical tissue in a nonfunctioning kidney due to arterial occlusion. This is due to enhancement of renal capsule and peripheral cortex from local collateral vessels.
▶ After acute renal infarction, the infarcted tissue parenchyma atrophies, leaving a cortical scar.

Management

▶ Anticoagulation

Further Reading

Kawashima A, Sandler CM, Ernst RD, Tamm EP, Goldman SM, Fishman EK. CT evaluation of renovascular disease. *Radiographics*. 2000;20(5):1321–1340.

History

▶ 60-year-old man with refractory hypertension

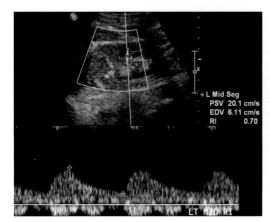

Figure 31.1

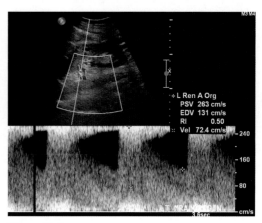

Figure 31.2

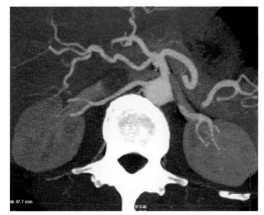

Figure 31.3

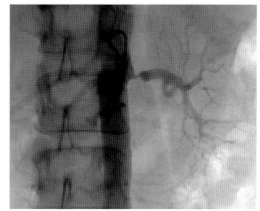

Figure 31.4

Case 31   Renal Artery Stenosis

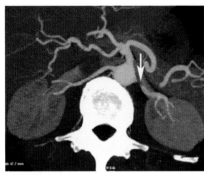
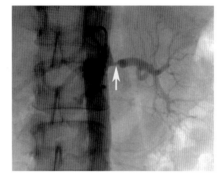

Figure 31.5   **Figure 31.6**

Findings

▶ Spectral Doppler waveform of a left interlobular artery (Figure 31.1) shows delayed upstroke (increased acceleration time), suggestive of upstream stenosis. Figure 31.2 shows elevated velocity at left main renal artery origin, which is causing aliasing of the arterial waveform.

▶ Axial maximum intensity projection reconstruction of CT angiogram (Figures 31.3 and 31.5) reveals severe focal stenosis of left main renal artery ostium (arrow in Figure 31.5).

▶ Catheter angiogram (Figures 31.4 and 31.6) confirms severe left main renal artery ostium stenosis (arrow in Figure 31.6).

Differential Diagnosis

▶ Atherosclerosis and fibromuscular dysplasia are the main causes of renal artery stenosis (RAS). Fibromuscular dysplasia can be excluded here as it occurs in a younger population, involves mid to distal renal artery, and has a typical string-of-pearls appearance on imaging. Narrowing of renal artery at ostium in an older patient, as seen here, is usually caused by atherosclerosis. Takayasu's arteritis (young females with aortic involvement) and type 1 neurofibromatosis (young patients with other characteristic stigmata) are rare causes of ostial and long-segment RAS.

Teaching Points

▶ Ninety percent of RAS is caused by atherosclerosis.
▶ Risk factors include older age, diabetes, renal dysfunction, extrarenal atherosclerotic disease, and smoking.
▶ Clinical presentation is with renal dysfunction and/or hypertension.
▶ Atherosclerotic stenosis involves ostium and proximal main renal artery.
▶ Renal Doppler sensitivity is 72%–92% for >70% diameter stenosis.
▶ Doppler features of main RAS include elevated peak velocity (>180–200 cm/s) and aliasing at site of stenosis, as well as main renal artery/aorta velocity ratio >3.5. Intrarenal arteries downstream of stenosis can have dampened waveform with delayed systolic upstroke.
▶ Sensitivity of CT angiogram in detecting RAS is 88%–96% and sensitivity of contrast MR angiogram is 88%–100%.
▶ Captopril renal scintigraphy provides functional assessment of renal perfusion and function. Its sensitivity and specificity are reduced in the presence of impaired renal function and bilateral stenoses.

Management

▶ Renal artery stenting

Further Reading

Kawashima A, Sandler CM, Ernst RD, Tamm EP, Goldman SM, Fishman EK. CT evaluation of renovascular disease. *Radiographics*. 2000;20(5):1321–1340.

History

▶ 45-year-old female with hypertension

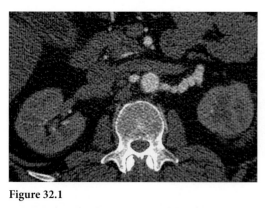

Figure 32.1

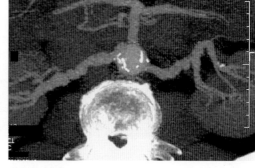

Figure 32.2

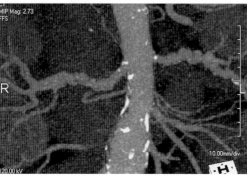

Figure 32.3

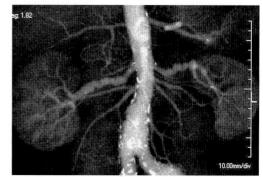

Figure 32.4

Case 32 Fibromuscular Dysplasia

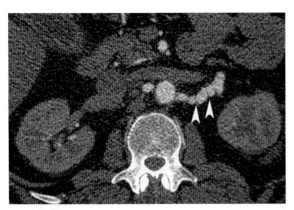

Figure 32.5

Findings

► Contrast-enhanced axial CT (Figure 32.1), axial and coronal maximum intensity projection (Figures 32.2 and 32.3), and volume rendered technique (VRT) reconstruction (Figure 32.4) images from a renal CT angiogram. A sequence of alternating outpouchings and indentations is present along the course of the renal artery (sparing the ostia), simulating beads threaded onto a string (arrowheads in Figure 32.5). Atherosclerotic calcification of the lower abdominal aorta and bilateral renal ostia is present (Figure 32.3).

Differential Diagnosis

► Differential diagnosis includes the two most common causes of renovascular hypertension: renal arterial atherosclerosis and fibromuscular dysplasia. Aortic calcification suggests the presence of atherosclerotic vascular disease. Renal arterial involvement by atherosclerosis typically causes stenosis of the renal ostia. Mild ostial calcification noted here does not cause significant narrowing, suggesting atherosclerosis is not the main pathology affecting the renal arteries. The string-of-pearls appearance of the bilateral renal arteries noted here is characteristic of fibromuscular dysplasia, which is the favored diagnosis.

Teaching Points

► Fibromuscular dysplasia is an idiopathic, nonatherosclerotic, noninflammatory disease that causes narrowing of small and medium-sized arteries.
► Fibromuscular dysplasia is the second most common cause of renovascular hypertension (10%) after renal artery stenosis (90%).
► It predominantly affects women in their fourth or fifth decades.
► Renal arterial involvement is present in 65%–70% of cases, but it can affect other arteries (carotid or vertebral involvement in 25%–30% of cases).
► Imaging features include involvement of mid to distal renal artery and its branches, string-of-pearls sign, aneurysms, and stenoses.
► String-of-pearls sign is seen only in medial hyperplasia subtype (which constitutes 85% of cases).
► Catheter angiogram remains the reference standard for diagnosis. CT and MR angiography have high accuracy. Ultrasound can miss stenotic segments if mid and distal arteries are not interrogated.

Management

► Percutaneous angioplasty without stenting

Further Reading

Beregi JP, Louvegny S, Gautier C, et al. Fibromuscular dysplasia of the renal arteries: comparison of helical CT angiography and arteriography. *AJR Am J Roentgenol.* 1999;172(1):27–34.

History

▶ 47-year-old female, status post left partial nephrectomy, presents with flank pain

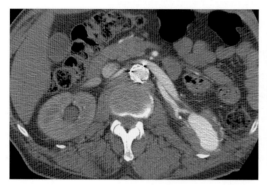

Figure 33.1

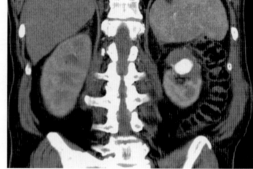

Figure 33.2

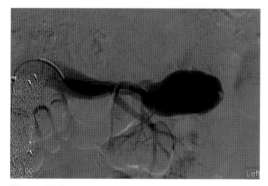

Figure 33.3

Case 33 Renal Arteriovenous Fistula

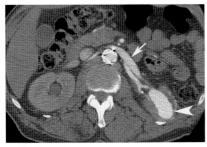

Figure 33.4

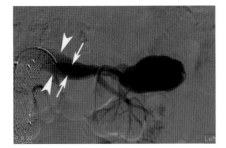

Figure 33.5

Findings

▶ Contrast-enhanced CT images (Figures 33.1 and 33.2) show a large dilated vascular structure (arrowhead in Figure 33.4) in the left kidney near the partial nephrectomy site. Large left renal artery and early opacification of left renal vein are noted (arrow in Figure 33.4). Adjacent parenchyma is poorly enhancing.

▶ Left renal angiogram reveals a large left renal artery (arrows in Figure 33.5) that is supplying the dilated vascular structure. Early filling of the left renal vein is seen (arrowheads in Figure 33.5).

Differential Diagnosis

▶ The dilated vascular structure in the left kidney with large feeding renal artery and early draining vein is diagnostic of an abnormal renal arteriovenous communication. History of recent renal intervention confirms this as an acquired renal arteriovenous fistula (AVF). The decreased parenchymal enhancement around the fistula is likely a combination of ischemia and post-surgical scarring. Cirsoid arteriovenous malformations, the most common congenital renal arteriovenous communication, consist of multiple small arteriovenous communications supplied by multiple arterial branches. Renal pseudoaneurysms occur following trauma; however, early filling of draining veins are not present, differentiating them from AVFs.

Teaching Points

▶ Congenital communications between the renal arterial and venous systems without intervening capillary bed are called renal arteriovenous malformations, while acquired abnormal communications are called renal AVFs. AVFs constitute 70%–80% of abnormal arteriovenous communications in kidney.

▶ Renal AVFs typically have a single enlarged feeding artery and a single enlarged draining vein.

▶ Penetrating trauma (biopsy, nephrostomy, stab injury) is the most common cause of renal AVF.

▶ Incidence of AVF is 5%–10% after renal biopsy. Most are asymptomatic and close spontaneously.

▶ Symptomatic AVFs cause flank pain, hematuria, hypertension, and heart failure.

▶ AVF is diagnosed on color Doppler by low-resistance flow in the supplying artery, high-velocity arterialized waveform in the draining vein, and turbulent high-velocity flow at the junction of the artery and vein.

Management

▶ Embolization or surgery

Further Reading

Kawashima A, Sandler CM, Ernst RD, Tamm EP, Goldman SM, Fishman EK. CT evaluation of renovascular disease. *Radiographics*. 2000;20(5):1321–1340.

History

▶ 25-year-old man with hematuria on physical exertion

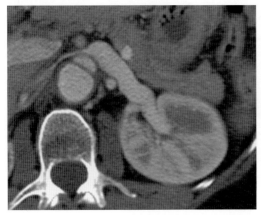

Figure 34.1

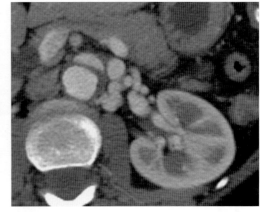

Figure 34.2

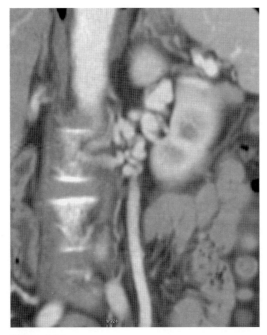

Figure 34.3

Case 34   Renal Vein Nutcracker Syndrome

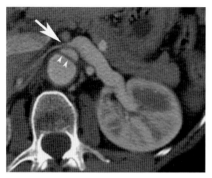

Figure 34.4

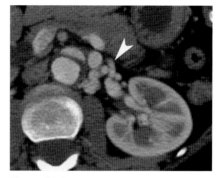

Figure 34.5

Findings

▶ Contrast-enhanced CT at the level of the left renal vein (Figure 34.1) shows abrupt narrowing and compression of the left renal vein between the superior mesenteric artery (SMA) and aorta (arrow in Figure 34.4). The vein is distended lateral to the narrowing and completely collapsed medial to it. Incidental aortic dissection is noted at this level (arrowheads in Figure 34.4).

▶ CT image just caudal to the renal vein (Figure 34.2) shows multiple collaterals around the renal hilum (arrowhead in Figure 34.5).

▶ Coronal reconstruction (Figure 34.3) depicts renal hilar collaterals and distended gonadal vein extending from the pelvis.

Differential Diagnosis

▶ The main diagnostic dilemma here is whether the narrowing of the renal vein between aorta and SMA is a normal incidental anatomic variant or represents entrapment of left renal vein in the mesoaortic angle with elevation of renal venous pressure (nutcracker syndrome). Significant distention of the renal vein proximal to the mesoaortic angle with complete collapse beyond it, development of multiple renal hilar collaterals, and distention of gonadal vein in this patient with hematuria suggest the diagnosis of nutcracker syndrome. Establishing the diagnosis of nutcracker syndrome is difficult, and renal venogram with pressure gradient measurement to demonstrate renal venous hypertension may be useful.

Teaching Points

▶ Nutcracker syndrome refers to the compression of the left renal vein between the SMA and aorta that results in renal venous hypertension.

▶ Clinical presentation may be with hematuria, flank pain, varicocele, or pelvic congestion syndrome.

▶ Correlation of imaging findings with clinical symptomatology is essential for diagnosis.

▶ Ratio of 4:1 of the distended to collapsed portions of the left renal vein is suggestive of nutcracker syndrome. Presence of venous collaterals supports the diagnosis.

▶ Doppler can demonstrate increase in the peak velocity ratio of the compressed part of the renal vein to the distended hilar part (ratio >4–5).

Management

▶ Interventions are controversial and limited to patients with persistent symptoms.

Further Reading
Kurklinsky AK, Rooke TW. Nutcracker phenomenon and nutcracker syndrome. *Mayo Clin Proc.* 2010;85(6):552–559.

History

▶ 42-year-old man with drop in hematocrit following extracorporeal shockwave lithotripsy (ESWL) for left renal stone disease

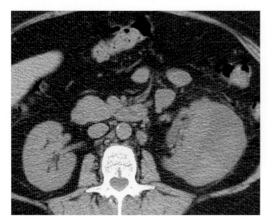

Figure 35.1

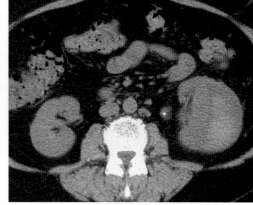

Figure 35.2

Case 35 Renal Subcapsular Hemorrhage

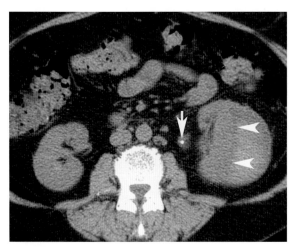

Figure 35.3

Findings

▶ Axial-unenhanced CT images (Figures 35.1–35.3) reveal a large high-attenuation collection abutting the left kidney, which exerts mass effect on the left renal parenchyma (arrowheads). A right proximal ureteral calculus (arrow) with adjacent ureteric wall thickening is noted.

Differential Diagnosis

▶ High attenuation of the collection is consistent with hemorrhage, which helps exclude other causes of perinephric fluid such as urinoma, lymphocele, or abscess. The collection is limited by the renal capsule and compresses the renal parenchyma, suggesting a subcapsular location. Subcapsular hematomas can be due to trauma, surgery, or underlying tumor. History of recent ESWL helps in establishing diagnosis of postoperative subcapsular hematoma with residual ureteral stone fragment in this patient. Follow-up imaging is performed in case of spontaneous hemorrhage to exclude underlying tumor.

Teaching Points

▶ Subcapsular and perinephric hematomas occur following trauma, renal surgery, and biopsy.
▶ Spontaneous hemorrhage into the subcapsular and perinephric space (Wunderlich syndrome) is due to underlying renal tumor in about 60% of cases. Angiomyolipoma is the underlying cause slightly more often than renal cell carcinoma. Other causes include vasculitis and underlying vascular malformation.
▶ In patients with spontaneous renal hemorrhage, repeat imaging is recommended after resolution of acute episode to evaluate for underlying neoplasm.
▶ Large, chronic subcapsular hematomas can reduce flow to the kidney and result in renin-mediated hypertension (Page kidney). Hypertension can develop days to even decades after the acute incident (mean 3 years).

Management

▶ Conservative management is recommended. Arterial embolization is required in life-threatening hemorrhage.

Further Reading

Katabathina VS, Katre R, Prasad SR, Surabhi VR, Shanbhogue AK, Sunnapwar A. Wunderlich syndrome: cross-sectional imaging review. *J Comput Assist Tomogr*. 2011;35(4):425–433.

History

▸ 40-year-old man with recurrent right flank pain

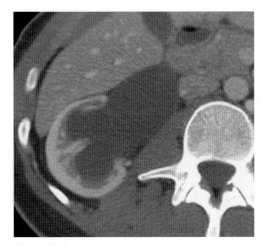

Figure 36.1

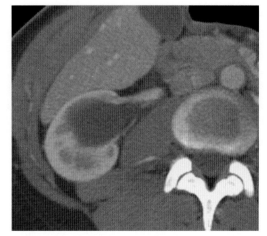

Figure 36.2

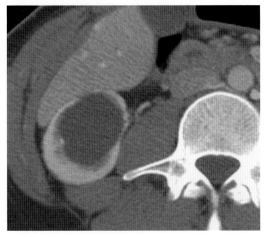

Figure 36.3

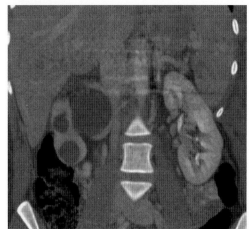

Figure 36.4

Case 36 Ureteropelvic Junction Obstruction with Crossing Vessel

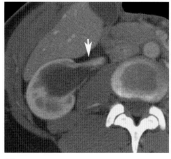 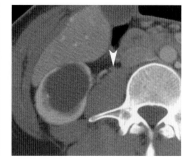 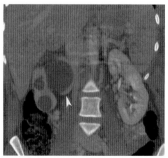

Figure 36.5   Figure 36.6   Figure 36.7

Findings

▶ Contrast-enhanced CT images (Figures 36.1–36.4) show severe dilation of the renal pelvis and collecting system. An accessory renal vein crosses the ureteropelvic junction (UPJ) anteriorly at the level of the obstruction (arrow in Figures 36.5 and 36.7). The ureter just distal to the crossing vein is normal in caliber (arrowhead in Figure 36.6).

Differential Diagnosis

▶ UPJ obstruction is caused by intrinsic muscular defect or acquired stricture or is associated with a crossing vessel. The close apposition of the crossing renal vein to the UPJ at the level of the obstruction supports the diagnosis in this patient.

Teaching Points

▶ Incidence of UPJ obstruction is 1 in 500 in neonates. It is much less common in adults, although the exact incidence is not known.

▶ Adults present with chronic back pain or acute renal colic. Ingestion of a large amount of fluid can cause excruciating pain due to renal pelvic distention. This may be accompanied by vomiting, hematuria, and general collapse (Dietl's crisis).

▶ Intrinsic muscular defect is almost always the underlying cause of neonatal UPJ obstruction. Adult UPJ obstruction is often caused by acquired stenosis (due to stone, infection, trauma).

▶ Crossing vessels may cause obstruction, exacerbate obstruction due to other cause, or just be "innocent bystanders." Crossing vessels, whether causal or incidental, are seen in 25%–50% of adult patients with UPJ.

▶ Identification of anterior and posterior crossing vessels (whether incidental or causative) during preoperative imaging is essential to prevent intraoperative hemorrhage and plan vasculopexy if required.

Management

▶ Using minimally invasive techniques such as endopyelotomy, an incision is made at UPJ to relieve obstruction. Crossing vessels are not visualized during the procedure, and risk of hemorrhage is higher.

▶ Open or laparoscopic pyeloplasty is favored in the presence of crossing vessels as they allow better visualization of vessels and can be combined with vasculopexy.

Further Reading
Grasso M, Caruso RP, Phillips CK. UPJ obstruction in the adult population: are crossing vessels significant? *Rev Urol.* 2001;3(1):42–45.

History

▶ 28-year-old man after motor vehicle accident

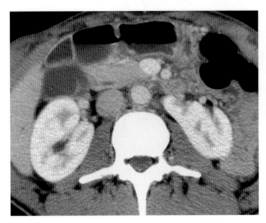

Figure 37.1

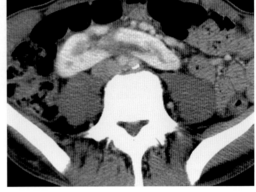

Figure 37.2

Case 37 Horseshoe Kidney with Laceration

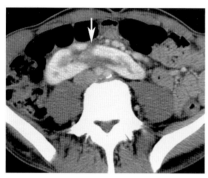

Figure 37.3

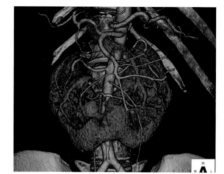

Figure 37.4

Findings

▶ Contrast-enhanced CT images (Figures 37.1–37.3) show fusion of the lower poles of both kidneys in the midline by an isthmus of functional renal parenchyma. A linear nonenhancing area with some stranding is present in the bridging enhancing renal parenchyma (arrow in Figure 37.3).

▶ Reconstructed CT image from a different patient (Figure 37.4) demonstrates the renal anatomy with midline fusion of the lower poles. Complex arterial supply of the kidney is noted.

Differential Diagnosis

▶ Fusion of the lower pole of both kidneys is diagnostic of horseshoe kidney. The linear nonenhancing area in the isthmus represents renal laceration in this patient with abdominal trauma.

Teaching Points

▶ Horseshoe kidney constitutes about 90% of renal fusion anomalies and is seen in <0.25% of the population.

▶ It occurs due to the fusion of each metanephric blastema during abnormal cell migration.

▶ Horseshoe kidney consists of two functional vertical kidneys on either side that are connected at their lower poles by an isthmus of functional parenchyma or, less commonly, by fibrotic tissue.

▶ The isthmus is generally located immediately below the origin of the inferior mesenteric artery, which prevents further ascension of the fused kidney.

▶ The arterial supply of a horseshoe kidney is often complex and includes branches from the aorta, iliac arteries, and inferior mesenteric artery.

▶ Horseshoe kidney is not protected by the rib cage and is vulnerable to blunt abdominal trauma. The midline isthmus can be forcefully compressed between the abdominal wall and vertebral body.

▶ Ureters have a high insertion into the renal pelvis and an angular course as they pass over the lower poles and isthmus. The abnormal course makes the upper ureters prone to obstruction.

▶ Obstruction at the ureteropelvic junction is present in 35% of patients. Stasis results in increased risk of infection and stone formation.

Management

▶ Management of complications

Further Reading

O'Brien J, Buckley O, Doody O, Ward E, Persaud T, Torreggiani W. Imaging of horseshoe kidneys and their complications. *J Med Imaging Radiat Oncol.* 2008;52(3):216–226.

History

▶ 63-year-old female with right flank pain

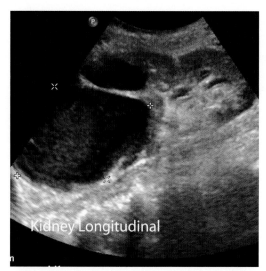

Figure 38.1

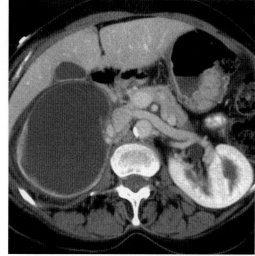

Figure 38.2

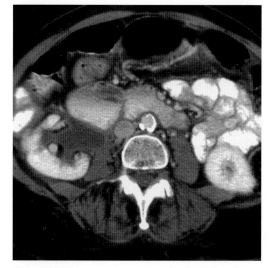

Figure 38.3

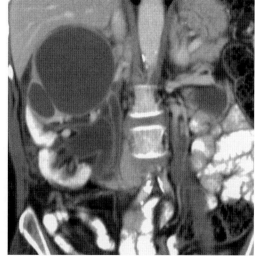

Figure 38.4

Case 38 Complete Duplex Collecting System/Ureter

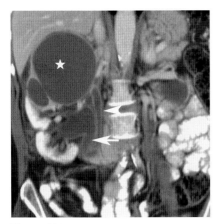

Figure 38.5

Findings

► Longitudinal renal ultrasound (Figure 38.1) shows a cystic structure replacing the right upper kidney. The lower aspect of the kidney appears normal.

► Contrast-enhanced CT images (Figures 38.2–38.4) confirm the right upper kidney is replaced by a cystic structure (asterisk Figure 38.5). The lower kidney has parenchymal scarring and mild pelvicalyceal dilation. Two right ureters are noted, with one draining the preserved lower kidney (arrow in Figure 38.5) and the other extending to the upper renal cystic sac (arrowhead in Figure 38.5).

Differential Diagnosis

► A duplex system is defined as a kidney with two pelvicalyceal systems associated with bifid or double ureters. Complete duplex systems have double ureters with two ureteric openings. The upper renal moiety ureteric opening is ectopic, located inferior and medial to the opening of the lower moiety ureter (Weigert–Meyer rule). The upper moiety ureter is prone to obstruction, while the lower moiety ureter is prone to reflux. In this patient, the upper renal cystic structure represents the hydronephrotic sac of the upper renal moiety drained by an obstructed ectopic ureter. The ectopic ureter may be associated with a ureterocele (not seen here). Parenchymal scarring and mild pelvicaliectasis in the lower moiety are due to reflux and associated infection.

Teaching Points

► Complete duplex systems are more often associated with reflux, obstruction, and renal scarring compared with incomplete duplication.

► In females, insertion of the ectopic ureter distal to the bladder neck sphincter mechanism can cause continuous dribbling incontinence.

► Ultrasound identifies obstruction and ureterocele. Voiding cystourethrogram assesses reflux, and renal scintigraphy evaluates function. Intravenous urogram (IVU), CT urography, or MR urography is used for anatomic evaluation.

► The obstructed upper pole moiety is often not opacified on IVU. This results in asymmetric reduction in the number of calyces and/or inferolateral displacement of lower pole collecting system (drooping lily sign).

Management

► Treatment of infection and relief of obstruction

Further Reading

Berrocal T, López-Pereira P, Arjonilla A, Gutiérrez J. Anomalies of the distal ureter, bladder, and urethra in children: embryologic, radiologic, and pathologic features. *Radiographics*. 2002;22(5):1139–1136.

History

▶ 46-year-old woman, 8 days post renal transplant with oliguria

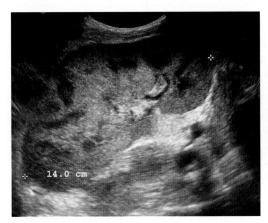

Figure 39.1

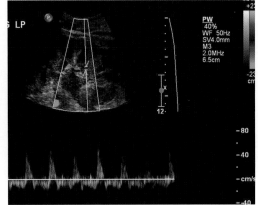

Figure 39.2

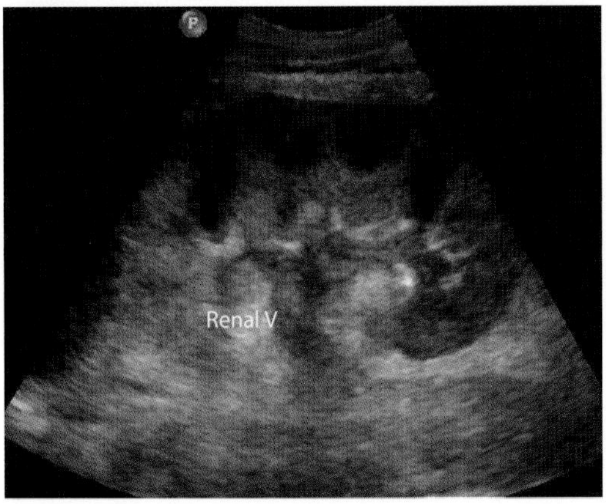

Figure 39.3

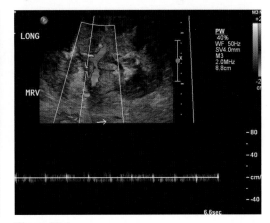

Figure 39.4

Transplant Renal Vein Thrombosis

Findings

► Grayscale ultrasound image (Figure 39.1) shows an enlarged (14 cm) echogenic transplant kidney. Spectral evaluation of segmental renal artery (Figure 39.2) reveals reversed diastolic flow. Grayscale evaluation of the main renal vein shows echogenic clot filling the lumen (Figure 39.3). No color flow or detectable spectral waveform is noted in the main renal vein (Figure 39.4).

Differential Diagnosis

► Enlargement of renal allograft is a nonspecific indicator of renal dysfunction and can be seen with rejection, acute tubular necrosis (ATN), or renal vein thrombosis. Reversed diastolic flow is an unusual finding noted in renal vein thrombosis, ATN, rejection, and allograft compression by perinephric hematoma. Although this finding is more frequently associated with ATN and acute rejection, renal vein thrombosis represents a more devastating entity that requires urgent intervention. The presence of renal enlargement and reversed diastolic flow in this patient triggered a more focused evaluation of the renal vein, which confirmed transplant renal vein thrombosis as the cause of the abnormal findings.

Teaching Points

► Reversed diastolic flow is seen in approximately 1% of post renal transplant patients.
► Reversed diastolic flow is sensitive but not specific for renal vein thrombosis. The majority of patients with this finding do not have renal vein thrombosis.
► Renal vein thrombosis usually presents in the first post-operative week.
► Clinically it manifests as oliguria and abdominal tenderness.
► Obstruction of the venous outflow results in increased arterial resistance, leading to diastolic reversal in the main renal and segmental arteries.
► Renal vein thrombosis is frequently associated with graft loss.

Management

► Urgent thrombectomy, if detected acutely

Further Reading
Lockhart ME, Wells CG, Morgan DE, Fineberg NS, Robbin ML. Reversed diastolic flow in the renal transplant: perioperative implications versus transplants older than 1 month. *AJR Am J Roentgenol.* 2008;190(3):65.

History

▶ 54-year-old male, 3 months post renal transplant with increasing serum creatinine

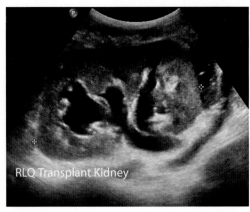

Figure 40.1

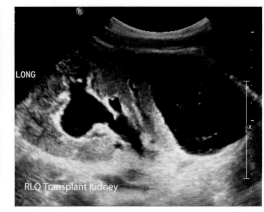

Figure 40.2

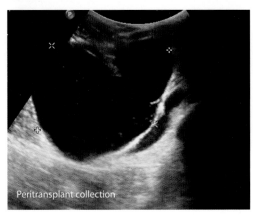

Figure 40.3

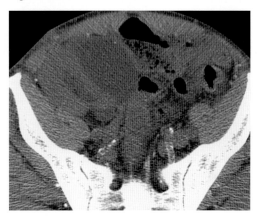

Figure 40.4

Case 40 Peritransplant Lymphocele

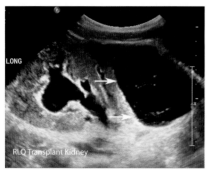

Figure 40.5

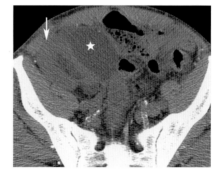

Figure 40.6

Findings

▶ Ultrasound images of the right lower quadrant reveal moderate transplant renal hydroureteronephrosis (Figure 40.1). A large collection with internal septa abuts the transplant kidney (Figure 40.2, arrows in Figure 40.5). Figure 40.3 shows the mildly complex peritransplant collection.

▶ Unenhanced CT image (Figure 40.4) confirms the ultrasound findings and demonstrates a fluid collection (asterisk in Figure 40.6) abutting and compressing the transplant kidney (arrow in Figure 40.6).

Differential Diagnosis

▶ A peritransplant collection may represent a hematoma, urinoma, lymphocele, or abscess. The time of presentation after surgery is indicative of the underlying etiology. Hematomas develop immediately after transplantation, are high attenuation on CT, and resolve over a few days. Urinomas and lymphoceles are similar on imaging but need to be differentiated due to different management algorithms. Urinomas usually develop early in the post-operative period, while lymphoceles often present 2 weeks to 6 months after transplantation. In this patient, presentation 3 months after transplantation favors a lymphocele, which was confirmed by aspiration. The transplant hydronephrosis noted here is secondary to compression and obstruction of the allograft by the lymphocele. Superinfection of any collection can result in abscess formation.

Teaching Points

▶ Lymphoceles develop due to disruption of lymphatics during surgery.

▶ Lymphoceles occur in 1%–26% of renal transplants; most are small and asymptomatic.

▶ Tense lymphoceles can cause graft dysfunction by direct pressure on the kidney, ureter, or vasculature.

▶ Urinomas develop due to urine leaks, often at the ureteric anastomosis.

▶ Fluid aspiration and analysis of creatinine level help differentiate urinoma from lymphocele. Infection can also be assessed.

▶ Renal scintigraphy can help identify a urine leak as well as assess for urinary obstruction.

Management

▶ Symptomatic lymphoceles can be managed by aspiration, drainage, sclerotherapy, or surgical drainage.

▶ Urinomas are managed by ureteric stenting and drainage of collection.

Further Reading
Richard HM. Perirenal transplant fluid collections. *Semin Intervent Radiol.* 2004;21(4):235–237.

History

▶ 40-year-old male, 5 days post-cadaveric renal transplant with delayed graft function

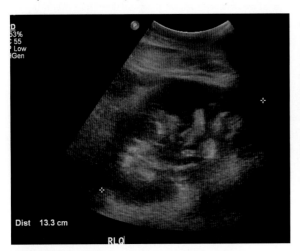

Figure 41.1

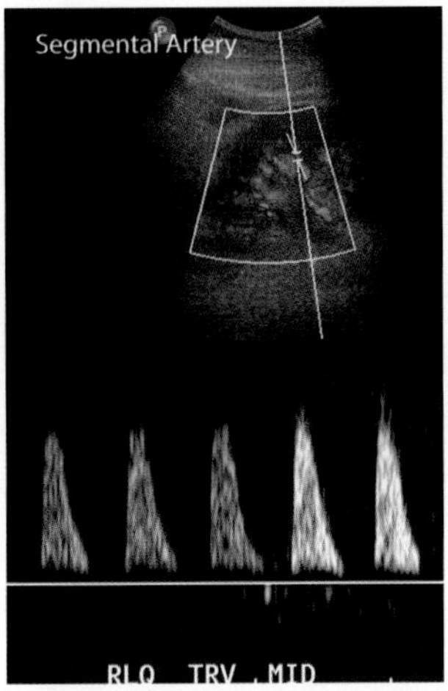

Figure 41.2

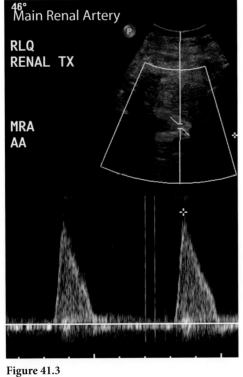

Figure 41.3

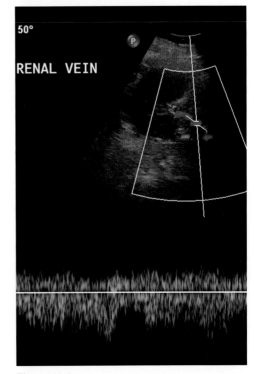

Figure 41.4

Case 41   Renal Transplant with Acute Tubular Necrosis

Findings

► Grayscale ultrasound image (Figure 41.1) shows an enlarged (13.3 cm) transplant kidney. Spectral tracing of a segmental artery (Figure 41.2) shows high-resistance waveform with absent diastolic flow (resistive index [RI] = 1.0). Main renal artery at the anastomosis (Figure 41.3) also has a high-resistance waveform with minimal end diastolic flow (RI > 0.9). Figure 41.4 shows a patent renal vein.

Differential Diagnosis

► High-resistance waveform (RI > 0.9) in renal allograft is a nonspecific indicator of graft dysfunction. It can be seen in acute tubular necrosis (ATN), acute and chronic rejection, renal vein thrombosis, and, occasionally, in cyclosporine toxicity. Demonstration of patent renal vein excludes renal vein thrombosis. The timeline of graft dysfunction after surgery is the best indicator of the underlying cause. Acute rejection rarely presents in the first few days after transplant. Rejection causes deterioration of graft function after the first week of transplant. ATN presents in the first few days after transplant with delayed function of the allograft. Although there is overlap in the timeline of ATN and acute rejection, delayed graft function in the first week, as seen in this case, is more compatible with ATN than acute rejection. Spontaneous function recovery after a few days confirmed the diagnosis.

Teaching Points

► Renal failure that persists after transplantation and requires dialysis in the first post-operative week is called delayed graft function. ATN is the most common cause of delayed graft function.
► ATN is common in cadaveric transplants and has a very low incidence in living donor recipients.
► ATN is caused by renal ischemia due to hypoperfusion, prolonged warm and cold ischemia times, and harvesting conditions.
► Graft function usually starts spontaneously within 14 days in patients with ATN.
► Presence of ATN makes detection of rejection difficult in post-transplant patients.
► If renal dysfunction persists, allograft biopsy may be necessary to differentiate between ATN and rejection

Management

► Supportive

Further Reading
Park SB, Kim JK, Cho KS. Complications of renal transplantation: ultrasonographic evaluation. *J Ultrasound Med.* 2007;26(5):615–633.

History

▶ 33-year-old male with incidental finding on abdominal CT imaging

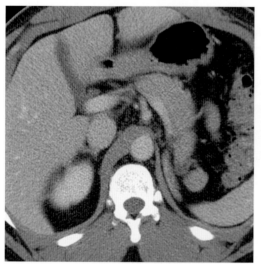

Figure 42.1

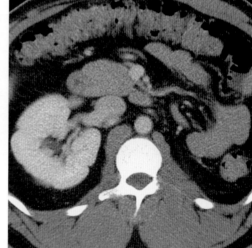

Figure 42.2

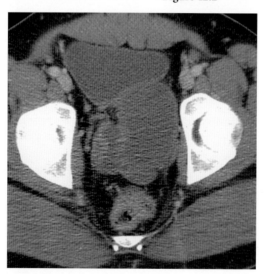

Figure 42.3

Case 42 Unilateral Renal Aplasia

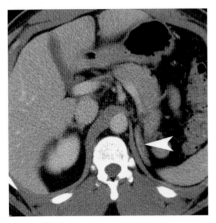
Figure 42.4

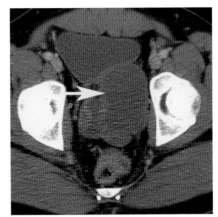
Figure 42.5

Findings

▶ Contrast-enhanced CT images (Figures 42.1–42.3) show an empty left renal fossa and a normal right kidney. A normally located but linear appearing left adrenal is present (arrowhead in Figure 42.4). A large cystic lesion is present posterior to the bladder in the expected region of the left seminal vesicle (arrow in Figure 42.5).

Differential Diagnosis

▶ Absence of left kidney in a patient without history of nephrectomy is diagnostic of congenital unilateral renal aplasia. Linear configuration of the left adrenal on the axial CT represents a discoid adrenal. The left pelvic cyst is compatible with a congenital seminal vesicle cyst, commonly seen in association with ipsilateral renal agenesis.

Teaching Points

▶ Normal adrenal glands have a triangular shape that forms due to indentation by the upper pole of the kidney. In the absence of renal development, adrenals assume a discoid morphology due to lack of local influence from the ipsilateral kidney.
▶ Unilateral renal agenesis occurs in 1 in 2000 births. The ipsilateral adrenal is present in more than 85% of patients.
▶ Bilateral renal agenesis is incompatible with life.
▶ In females, renal agenesis is associated with vaginal atresia, vaginal septum, and uterine aplasia.
▶ In males, renal agenesis is associated with ipsilateral congenital unilateral seminal vesicle cyst, cryptorchidism, hypospadias, and absence of testis.

Management

▶ Usually asymptomatic

Further Reading

Livingston L, Larsen CR. Seminal vesicle cyst with ipsilateral renal agenesis. *AJR Am J Roentgenol.* 2000;175(1):177–180.

History

▶ 51-year-old female on treatment for bipolar mood disorder for last 3 years

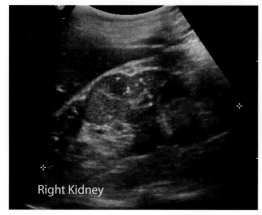

Figure 43.1

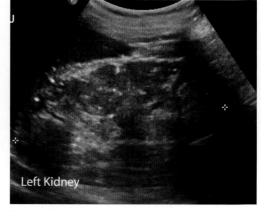

Figure 43.2

Case 43 Lithium Nephrotoxicity

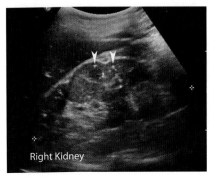 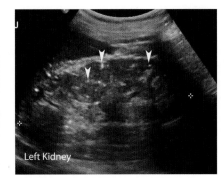

Figure 43.3   **Figure 43.4**

Findings

▶ Ultrasound images of both kidneys (Figures 43.1 and 43.2) reveal multiple nonshadowing tiny echogenic foci throughout both renal cortex and medulla (arrowheads in Figures 43.3 and 43.4).

Differential Diagnosis

▶ Multiple nonshadowing tiny echogenic foci in the cortex and medulla of both kidneys in a patient being treated for bipolar disorder are characteristic of lithium nephrotoxicity. Renal calculi also appear as echogenic foci in the kidneys but show posterior acoustic shadowing and usually do not have the diffuse distribution throughout the renal cortex and medulla noted here.

Teaching Points

▶ Nephrotoxicity is a common adverse effect of lithium treatment.
▶ Risk of nephrotoxicity increases with duration of treatment.
▶ Lithium nephrotoxicity causes formation of tiny 1- to 2-mm cysts scattered in the cortex and medulla.
▶ Echogenic foci scattered in the renal parenchyma likely represent microcysts below the resolution of ultrasound, not calcifications.
▶ Ultrasound may also demonstrate numerous small renal cysts in patients with lithium nephrotoxicity.
▶ Microcysts are identified as T2 hyperintense foci on MRI.

Management

▶ Discontinuation of drug and consideration of alternative therapy

Further Reading

Karaosmanoglu AD, Butros SR, Arellano R. Imaging findings of renal toxicity in patients on chronic lithium therapy. *Diagn Interv Radiol*. 2013;19(4):299–303.

History

▶ Two 50 and 53-year-old male patients with gross hematuria

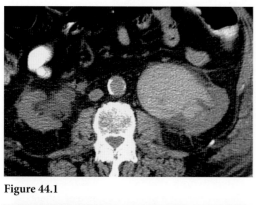

Figure 44.1

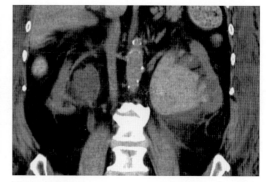

Figure 44.2

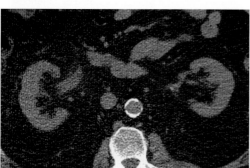

Figure 44.3

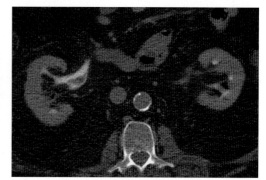

Figure 44.4

Case 44 Collecting System Hemorrhage

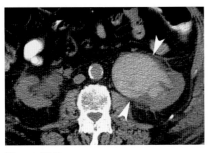

Figure 44.5

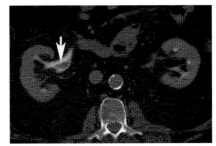

Figure 44.6

Findings

▶ Unenhanced CT images (Figures 44.1–44.2) reveal high-attenuation material distending the left renal pelvis and collecting system (arrowheads in Figure 44.5). Incidental note is made of atrophic right kidney.

▶ Figures 44.3 and 44.4 are unenhanced and nephropyelographic-phase CT images from a different patient. No lesion is discernible on the unenhanced scan. Nephropyelographic phase shows a linear filling defect with tapering edges in the right renal pelvis (arrow in Figure 44.6).

Differential Diagnosis

▶ Differential diagnosis in both patients includes blood clot in the collecting system and transitional cell carcinoma. Transitional cell carcinoma is soft-tissue attenuation and enhances after contrast administration, while blood clot is usually high attenuation and does not enhance. In the first patient, the high attenuation within the collecting system on the unenhanced image is typical of a large clot. In the second patient, the diagnosis is more difficult as the small right renal pelvic lesion is not hyperdense on the unenhanced scan. On the nephropyelographic phase, the lesion is surrounded by high-attenuation contrast, making assessment of enhancement difficult. The filling defect, however, has a linear configuration with tapering angular edges at the point of contact with the urothelium. It is largely separated from the urothelium by intervening contrast. This configuration favors a retracting blood clot over transitional cell carcinoma.

Teaching Points

▶ Blood clots in the collecting system can be seen in patients with hematuria.

▶ Hemorrhage may be secondary to infection, anticoagulation, or vascular malformation; iatrogenic; or due to underlying tumor.

▶ Large blood clot may mask a small underlying tumor.

▶ MRI may show high T1 signal intensity of the clot.

Management

▶ Treat the underlying cause of hematuria

Further Reading

O'Connor OJ, Fitzgerald E, Maher MM. Imaging of hematuria. *AJR Am J Roentgenol.* 2010;195(4):W263–267.

Section II   Retroperitoneum

History

▶ 40-year-old man with backache

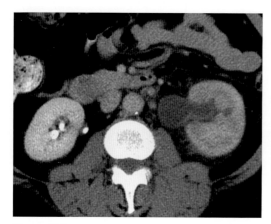

Figure 45.1

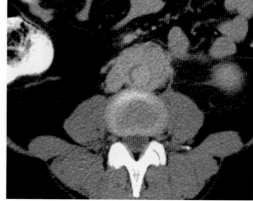

Figure 45.2

Case 45 Retroperitoneal Fibrosis

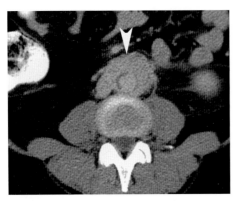

Figure 45.3

Findings

▶ Contrast-enhanced CT images (Figures 45.1 and 45.2) show confluent soft tissue (arrowhead in Figure 45.3) surrounding the infrarenal aorta. The soft tissue is most prominent anterior and lateral to the aorta without anterior displacement of aorta. There is hydronephrosis, delayed enhancement, and stranding around the left kidney secondary to ureteric obstruction.

Differential Diagnosis

▶ Differential diagnosis of confluent soft tissue proliferation around the abdominal aorta includes idiopathic or secondary retroperitoneal fibrosis (RPF) and confluent retroperitoneal lymphoma. Anterior displacement of aorta, additional lymphadenopathy, and perirenal extension are features of lymphoma. Absence of these features would favor RPF but is not diagnostic. Medial ureteral bowing (not easily identified on CT) and pelvic extension are more common in RPF. Diagnosis of idiopathic RPF was confirmed by biopsy.

Teaching Points

▶ RPF is characterized by plaque-like fibrotic proliferative reaction. It usually starts around the aortic bifurcation and iliac arteries and extends through the retroperitoneum to involve the ureters.
▶ Two-thirds of RPF cases are idiopathic and likely autoimmune in origin. It is associated with fibrosing conditions such as Reidel's thyroiditis, sclerosing cholangitis, and orbital pseudotumor.
▶ Idiopathic RPF typically occurs in those aged 40–60 years, with male preponderance.
▶ RPF can be secondary to inflammatory aortic aneurysms, desmoplastic reaction to disseminated malignancy, drugs, or radiation. Malignant RPF is caused by small retroperitoneal neoplastic foci, which elicit a desmoplastic response.
▶ On imaging, enhancement is present during chronic active phase of inflammation and decreases in mature fibrotic stage.
▶ RPF tethers the aorta and inferior vena cava to underlying vertebrae and does not elevate them. However, RPF secondary to malignancy can have soft tissue between the aorta and vertebra.
▶ Differentiating idiopathic and malignant RPF on percutaneous biopsy is challenging. In malignant RPF, few malignant cells may be dispersed in dense fibrotic tissue, and multiple core biopsy specimens are obtained to limit undersampling.

Management

▶ Identification and treatment/removal of underlying cause, if any
▶ Steroids and immunotherapy for idiopathic RPF

Further Reading
Cronin CG, Lohan DG, Blake MA, Roche C, McCarthy P, Murphy JM. Retroperitoneal fibrosis: a review of clinical features and imaging findings. *AJR Am J Roentgenol.* 2008;191(2):423–431.

History

▶ 50-year-old man with backache

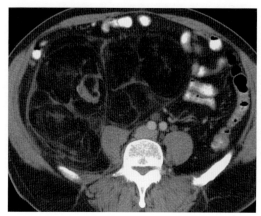

Figure 46.1

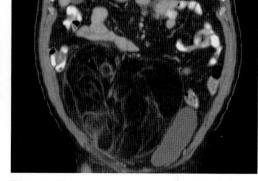

Figure 46.2

Case 46 Retroperitoneal Liposarcoma

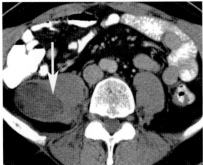

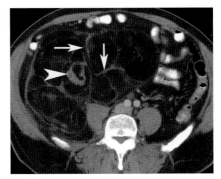

Figure 46.3

Figure 46.4

Findings

► Contrast-enhanced CT images (Figures 46.1 and 46.2) show a large predominantly fat-attenuation retroperitoneal mass. Multiple septa (arrows in Figure 46.4) and a nodular component (arrowhead in Figure 46.4) are noted.

► Figure 46.3, which is from a different patient, shows a heterogeneous, low-attenuation retroperitoneal mass (arrow) involving the psoas muscle.

Differential Diagnosis

► Differential diagnosis of fat-containing retroperitoneal lesion includes liposarcoma, lipoma, large exophytic renal angiomyolipoma, and teratoma. Absence of a fatty renal cortical defect or large intratumoral vessels from the kidney excludes renal angiomyolipoma. Retroperitoneal teratoma is excluded as it presents in children/young adults and is characterized by the presence of calcification and a cystic component (often with fat fluid level). Lipomas are exceedingly rare in the retroperitoneum, and this diagnosis is often due to undersampling of a liposarcoma. Large size (>10 cm) and presence of septa/nodular component in this fatty lesion favor diagnosis of malignant liposarcoma over a benign lipoma. Predominance of mature fat suggests it is a well-differentiated subtype of liposarcoma. Presence of solid components in such a lesion would raise suspicion of dedifferentiation into more aggressive tumor. Pleomorphic liposarcomas are solid, heterogeneous soft tissue masses that often do not contain any fat on imaging.

► Heterogeneous hypoattenuating mass with interspersed subtle areas of fat attenuation seen in Figure 46.3 is suggestive of a myxoid liposarcoma. These do not contain large amounts of mature fat but have distribution of fat and soft tissue, resulting in low attenuation on CT.

Teaching Points

► Liposarcomas constitute 35% of all malignant retroperitoneal soft tissue tumors in adult patients.

► They are large, slow-growing tumors that present in the sixth and seventh decades.

► Well-differentiated liposarcoma is the most common subtype. These do not metastasize but recur after excision.

► Dedifferentiation results in more aggressive tumor with metastatic potential.

► On MRI, myxoid liposarcomas have low T1 and high T2 signals due to the myxoid matrix, resulting in pseudocystic appearance. Enhancement helps differentiate them from cysts.

Management

► Surgical excision

Further Reading

Craig WD, Fanburg-Smith JC, Henry LR, Guerrero R, Barton JH. Fat-containing lesions of the retroperitoneum: radiologic-pathologic correlation. *Radiographics.* 2009;29(1):261–290.

History

▶ 40-year-old man with severe hypertension and elevated urinary metanephrines

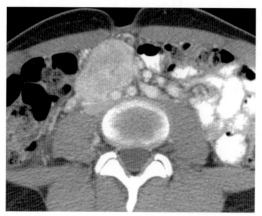

Figure 47.1

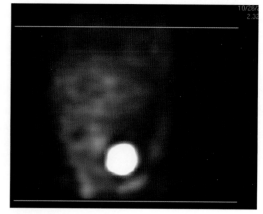

Figure 47.2

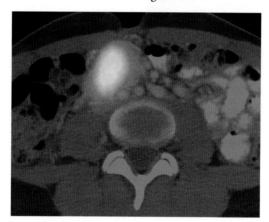

Figure 47.3

Case 47 Paraganglioma

Findings

▶ Contrast-enhanced CT imaging (Figure 47.1) shows a large, inhomogeneous hyperenhancing mass at the aortic bifurcation.

▶ I-123 metaiodobenzylguanidine (MIBG) scintigram shows focal area of intense radiotracer uptake in the mid abdomen (Figure 47.2).

▶ Fusion of MIBG and CT images shows that the intense activity corresponds to the hypervascular mass (Figure 47.3).

Differential Diagnosis

▶ In a patient with hypertension and elevated urinary metanephrines, presence of a hyperenhancing mass at aortic bifurcation is highly suggestive of a catecholamine-secreting paraganglioma arising from organ of Zuckerkandl. Intense MIBG uptake confirms this diagnosis. A mesenteric carcinoid metastasis can be hyperenhancing on CT and have MIBG uptake but will have different clinical and biochemical presentation of serotonin excess.

Teaching Points

▶ Paragangliomas are tumors that arise from paraganglia, which are distributed from the skull base to the pelvis. Tumors of paraganglia of adrenal medulla are called pheochromocytomas.

▶ Abdominal paragangliomas have predilection for organ of Zuckerkandl, which is a prominent collection of paraganglia near the origin of the inferior mesenteric artery.

▶ Paragangliomas commonly occur in the fourth and fifth decades without any sex predilection.

▶ They can be associated with type 1 neurofibromatosis, multiple endocrine neoplasia syndrome, and von Hippel–Lindau syndrome.

▶ Catecholamine hypersecretion is common in the thorax and retroperitoneal paragangliomas but not head and neck paragangliomas.

▶ Catecholamine production results in symptoms such as headache, palpitations, and excessive sweating.

▶ MIBG, a norepinephrine analogue, is taken up avidly by paragangliomas and pheochromocytomas.

▶ MIBG labeled with I-123 or I-131 has a very high specificity (95%–100%) for detecting paragangliomas. Sensitivity of MIBG is lower (85%).

▶ Paragangliomas enhance intensely after contrast administration due to hypervascularity.

▶ On T2 imaging, paragangliomas are hyperintense but often heterogeneous due to hemorrhage.

Management

▶ Surgical excision

Further Reading
Lee KY, Oh YW, Noh HJ, et al. Extraadrenal paragangliomas of the body: imaging features. *AJR Am J Roentgenol.* 2006;187(2):492–504.

History

▶ 60-year-old man with weight loss

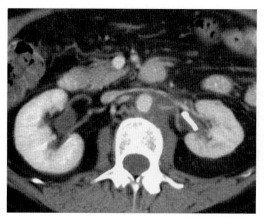

Figure 48.1

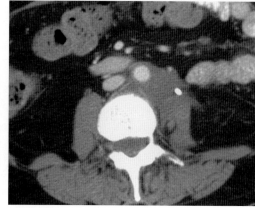

Figure 48.2

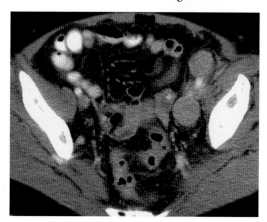

Figure 48.3

Case 48 Retroperitoneal Lymphoma

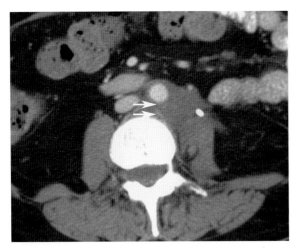

Figure 48.4

Findings

▶ Contrast-enhanced CT images (Figures 48.1–48.3) show homogeneous, confluent, hypoenhancing retroperitoneal soft tissue encasing and anteriorly displacing the aorta (floating aorta, arrows in Figure 48.4). The mass extends to the left renal hilum and encases the left renal artery and ureter (stent in place). Additional bulky left iliac lymphadenopathy is noted in Figure 48.3.

Differential Diagnosis

▶ Differential diagnosis includes lymphoma, retroperitoneal fibrosis, and retroperitoneal sarcoma. Retroperitoneal sarcomas are large heterogeneously enhancing tumors and can be excluded. Retroperitoneal lymphoma usually has discrete enlarged lymph nodes but may present as confluent soft tissue encasing the aorta. The elevation of the aorta by the soft tissue, as noted here, is a feature of lymphoma. It is unusual (although possible) for retroperitoneal fibrosis to do this. Retroperitoneal fibrosis usually involves the lower aorta and iliac, while confluent lymphoma tends to have more cranial and perirenal extension. Additional pelvic lymphadenopathy, as noted in this patient, helps clinch the diagnosis of lymphoma over retroperitoneal fibrosis.

Teaching Points

▶ Lymphoma is the most common retroperitoneal malignancy.
▶ Non-Hodgkin lymphoma presents as a retroperitoneal mass in 14% of cases.
▶ Abdominal Hodgkin lymphoma often involves the spleen and spreads to contiguous lymph nodes, while non-Hodgkin lymphoma involves discontinuous nodal groups and extranodal sites.
▶ Lymphoma is usually homogeneous and mildly enhancing on CT.
▶ Calcification and necrosis are unusual before therapy.
▶ Lymphomatous masses are usually hypoechoic on ultrasound.
▶ Lymphoma is isointense on T1-weighted imaging and iso- to hyperintense on T2-weighted imaging.
▶ Post-therapy fibrotic residual masses may persist in the absence of viable disease. Uptake on fluorodeoxyglucose positron emission tomography is an indicator of residual viable disease.

Management

▶ Chemotherapy or radiation

Further Reading
Rajiah P, Sinha R, Cuevas C, Dubinsky TJ, Bush WH Jr, Kolokythas O. Imaging of uncommon retroperitoneal masses. *Radiographics*. 2011;31(4):949–976.

History

▶ 65-year-old woman with flank pain

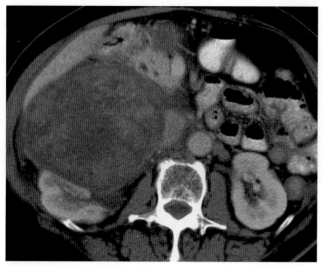

Figure 49.1

Case 49 Retroperitoneal Soft Tissue Sarcoma

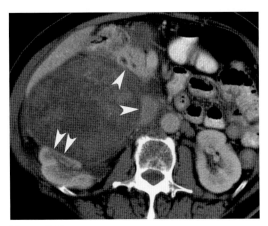

Figure 49.2

Findings

▶ Contrast-enhanced CT imaging (Figure 49.1) shows a large, heterogeneously enhancing mass with necrosis that displaces the pancreas anteriorly, kidney posteriorly, and inferior vena cava medially (arrowheads in Figure 49.2). The mass has a smooth broad interface with adjacent structures.

Differential Diagnosis

▶ The first step in creating a differential diagnosis is to determine the organ or compartment of origin. This neoplasm displaces the pancreas anteriorly, suggesting a retroperitoneal location. A tumor in the retroperitoneum can arise from a retroperitoneal organ or be a primary retroperitoneal tumor. In this patient, the abutting organs have crescentic deformation and smooth, rounded edges, rather than beaked edges at the interface with the mass. This is characteristic of a primary retroperitoneal tumor. When a mass deforms the edge of an adjacent organ into a beak shape, it is likely that the mass arose from that organ (beak sign).

▶ Differential diagnosis of primary retroperitoneal neoplasm includes mesodermal neoplasms, neurogenic tumors, and lymphoma. Lymphoma is less likely here as it is usually homogeneous, mildly enhancing, and associated with other lymphadenopathy. Neurogenic tumor is unlikely as they occur in younger patients and usually have paravertebral (and not perirenal) location. Among common retroperitoneal mesodermal tumors, most types of liposarcoma can be excluded due to the lack of macroscopic fat. Leiomyosarcomas, malignant fibrous histiocytoma, and other rarer sarcomas cannot be differentiated on imaging and all are possible. Leiomyosarcoma was diagnosed on histopathology.

Teaching Points

▶ Leiomyosarcoma (28%) and malignant fibrous histiocytoma (19%) are the second and third most common retroperitoneal sarcomas; liposarcoma is the most common. Rhabdomyosarcoma, fibrosarcoma, and angiosarcoma are rare mesodermal sarcomas.

▶ Leiomyosarcoma is more frequent in females, and malignant fibrous histiocytoma is more frequent in males.

▶ Most soft tissue sarcomas are large at presentation.

▶ On imaging, heterogeneous enhancement, necrosis, and cystic degeneration are common.

▶ Extensive vascular involvement, peritoneal implants, and distant metastatic disease suggest unresectability. Regional lymphadenopathy is uncommon (4%).

Management

▶ Complete surgical excision, when possible, is the most important prognostic factor.

Further Reading

Goenka AH, Shah SN, Remer EM. Imaging of the retroperitoneum. *Radiol Clin North Am*. 2012;50(2):333–355, vi.

History

▶ 38-year-old man with human immunodeficiency virus infection and fever

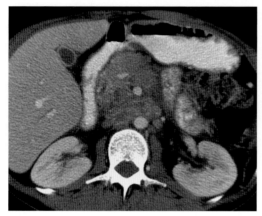

Figure 50.1

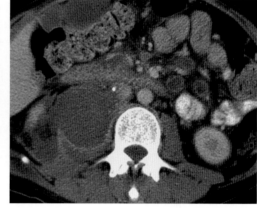

Figure 50.2

Case 50 Tuberculous Lymphadenopathy

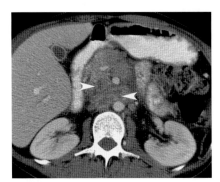

Figure 50.3

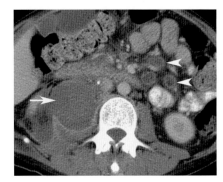

Figure 50.4

Findings

▶ Contrast-enhanced CT images (Figures 50.1 and 50.2) show multiple enlarged retroperitoneal peripancreatic and mesenteric lymph nodes with central low attenuation (arrowheads in Figures 50.3 and 50.4). A large rim-enhancing collection is present in the right psoas muscle (arrow in Figure 50.4).

Differential Diagnosis

▶ In a patient with human immunodeficiency virus infection (HIV), differential diagnosis of lymphadenopathy with central low attenuation includes tuberculosis, mycobacterium avium-intracellulare (MAC) infection, fungal infection, necrotic metastatic lymphadenopathy, and Whipple's disease. The last three diagnoses cannot account for the psoas abscess seen in this patient and are therefore unlikely. Kaposi's sarcoma and lymphoma, the two malignancies associated with HIV infection, cause uniform-attenuation, not low-attenuation, lymphadenopathy prior to therapy. Whipple's disease does not occur with increased frequency in HIV patients. Tuberculosis and MAC are common infections in HIV patients. Both infections cause low-attenuation, centrally necrotic lymphadenopathy and can have associated psoas abscess formation. Although it is not possible to distinguish between the two infections without tissue sampling, tuberculous lymph nodes are much more likely to have low-attenuation centers than MAC infection. Psoas abscess is also more commonly associated with tuberculous infection.

Teaching Points

▶ Lymphadenopathy is the most common manifestation of abdominal tuberculosis on CT.
▶ Lymph modes have low-attenuation centers in 40%–70% of patients. This represents central caseous necrosis in the lymph nodes.
▶ Lymph nodes may coalesce to form confluent masses.
▶ Tuberculosis commonly involves peripancreatic and mesenteric lymph nodes. Most patients with retroperitoneal lymph nodes have other concomitant sites of lymphadenopathy.
▶ Calcification can be seen in tuberculous lymph nodes.
▶ Involvement of the psoas muscle is often secondary to spread from spinal infection.

Management

▶ Drain psoas abscess percutaneously
▶ Anti-tuberculous drug therapy

Further Reading
Suri S, Gupta S, Suri R. Computed tomography in abdominal tuberculosis. *Br J Radiol.* 1999;72(853):92–98.

History

▶ 43-year-old female (Figures 51.1 and 51.2) and 50-year-old male (Figures 51.3 and 51.4) with incidental retroperitoneal lesions

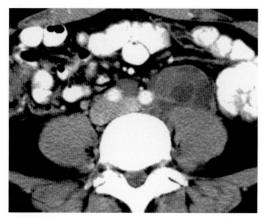

Figure 51.1

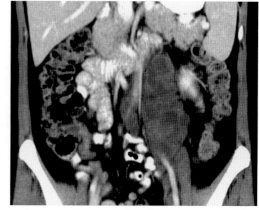

Figure 51.2

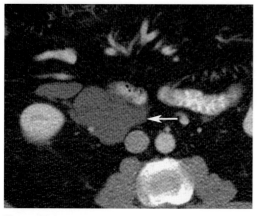

Figure 51.3

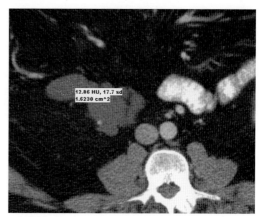

Figure 51.4

Case 51 Retroperitoneal Lymphangioma

Findings

▶ Contrast-enhanced CT images (Figures 51.1 and 51.2) show an elongated left periaortic retroperitoneal lesion with prominent cystic component and mildly enhancing thick septations.

▶ Figures 51.3 and 51.4 are CT images from a different patient. A multilocular, nonenhancing, fluid-attenuation (12 HU) cystic retroperitoneal lesion is present. The lesion extends medially between the inferior vena cava and adjacent bowel loop (arrow in Figure 3) and also insinuates around mesenteric vessels.

Differential Diagnosis

▶ Differential diagnosis includes cystic degeneration in a solid retroperitoneal tumor, necrosis related to therapy in a solid tumor, and primary retroperitoneal cystic lesions such as lymphangioma or cystic teratoma. Shwannomas and paragangliomas are retroperitoneal neurogenic tumors that can undergo cystic degeneration. Necrosis of solid retroperitoneal tumors following chemotherapy can also result in a cystic appearance. Cystic teratomas are identified by the presence of fat and calcification in addition to cystic component. Retroperitoneal lymphangiomas are benign unilocular or multilocular cysts and often have an elongated shape. The multilocular, elongated cystic retroperitoneal lesion in Figures 51.1 and 51.2, is consistent with the diagnosis of retroperitoneal lymphangioma. The enhancement and apparent soft tissue component noted are likely secondary to previous hemorrhage or infection.

▶ Figures 51.3 and 51.4, from a different patient, show a multilocular cystic retroperitoneal lesion that insinuates along tissue planes. This is also an example of a retroperitoneal lymphangioma. The lack of enhancement noted here is more typical of a lymphangioma that has not been complicated by hemorrhage or infection.

Teaching Points

▶ Lymphangiomas are benign developmental lesions of lymphovascular origin.

▶ They most often occur in the neck. Retroperitoneal lymphangiomas constitute <1% of all lymphangiomas.

▶ Lymphangiomas are the most common primary retroperitoneal cystic tumor.

▶ Lymphangiomas are thin-walled cystic masses that contain serous, chylous, or hemorrhagic fluid.

▶ Presence of hemorrhage or infection can give a more solid appearance. Walls and septa can enhance after contrast administration.

▶ Lymphangiomas tend to insinuate along tissue planes and traverse anatomic compartments.

Management

▶ No intervention needed if asymptomatic

Further Reading
Levy AD, Cantisani V, Miettinen M. Abdominal lymphangiomas: imaging features with pathologic correlation. *AJR Am J Roentgenol.* 2004;182(6):1485–1491.

History

▶ 56-year-old female with weight loss

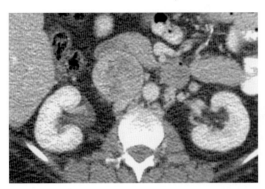

Figure 52.1

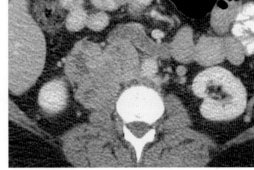

Figure 52.2

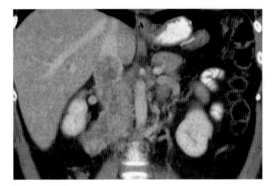

Figure 52.3

Case 52 Inferior Vena Cava Leiomyosarcoma

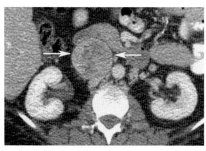 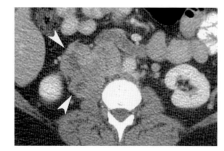

Figure 52.4   **Figure 52.5**

Findings

▶ Contrast-enhanced CT images (Figures 52.1–52.3) show a large, heterogeneously enhancing mass expanding the inferior vena cava (IVC; arrows in Figure 52.4). Extraluminal extension beyond the IVC is present (arrowheads in Figure 52.5).

Differential Diagnosis

▶ Bland thrombus is the most common filling defect in the IVC. Enhancement within the IVC mass excludes bland thrombus and confirms a neoplastic process. Large size and extraluminal extension suggest an aggressive neoplasm. Vascular invasion by primary malignancy of kidney, liver, or adrenal is the most common cause of enhancing tumor within the IVC. The primary lesion is obvious in these cases, and no such lesion is present in this patient. Malignant retroperitoneal sarcomas are aggressive tumors and can secondarily involve the IVC. Such lesions tend to displace the IVC, not expand it, making the diagnosis less likely. Expansion of the IVC noted here suggests the origin of the tumor is within the IVC. This is characteristic of primary IVC leiomyosarcoma, which is the favored diagnosis.

Teaching Points

▶ IVC leiomyosarcomas are rare malignant vascular tumors most frequently seen in the sixth decade with a female preponderance.

▶ Presenting symptoms are nonspecific and include abdominal pain, weight loss, dyspnea, edema and Budd Chiari syndrome.

▶ Location of tumor (middle, lower, or upper third of the IVC) affects symptomatology and ease of resection.

▶ IVC leiomyosarcomas can be completely intraluminal or have an extraluminal component.

▶ Prognosis is poor; the 10-year survival rate is 14%.

Management

▶ Surgical resection and consideration of systemic therapy

Further Reading

Ganeshalingam S, Rajeswaran G, Jones RL, Thway K, Moskovic E. Leiomyosarcomas of the inferior vena cava: diagnostic features on cross-sectional imaging. *Clin Radiol*. 2011;66(1):50–56.

History

▶ 37-year-old woman, 8 weeks post aortic graft surgery

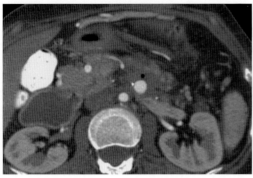

Figure 53.1

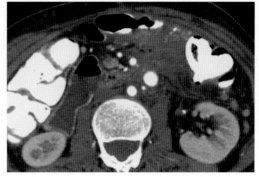

Figure 53.2

Case 53 Aortic Perigraft Infection with Colonic Fistula

Formation

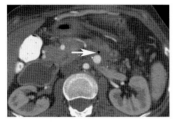 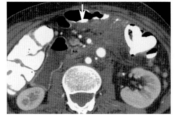 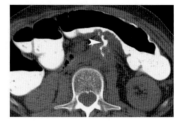

Figure 53.3   Figure 53.4   Figure 53.5

Findings

▶ Contrast-enhanced CT images (Figures 53.1 and 53.2) reveal exuberant soft tissue around aortic bypass graft with a focus of gas (arrow in Figure 53.3). Adjacent colon wall thickening is present (arrow in Figure 53.4).

▶ CT image obtained after 4 weeks (Figure 53.5) reveals oral contrast tracking from the colon to the aortic graft (arrowhead).

▶ The diminutive native aorta is secondary to underlying large vessel vasculitis.

Differential Diagnosis

▶ Persistent perigraft soft-tissue or fluid attenuation can indicate infection or represent normal post-operative change. Post-operative perigraft soft tissue or fluid is usually seen only during the immediate post-surgical period but may persist for 3 months. Perigraft gas is rare beyond the first post-operative week, and no air should be present at 3–4 weeks. In this patient, the presence of perigraft air at 8 weeks is almost pathognomonic of an infectious process. Although gas-forming organisms can cause perigraft gas, this finding strongly indicates presence of an aortoenteric fistula that is complicating the infection. Bowel wall thickening also favors this diagnosis.

Teaching Points

▶ Prosthetic graft infection occurs in 1.3%–6% of patients with graft insertion but has a high mortality (25%–75%). Aortoenteric fistula is a complication of graft infection.

▶ Seventy percent of graft infections manifest after the first year. In acute infections (within 4 months of surgery), patients are acutely ill with fever. Symptoms are often nonspecific in late-onset infection and include back pain, malaise, and gastrointestinal bleeding.

▶ CT has sensitivity of 94% and specificity of 85% for graft infection when the criteria of perigraft fluid, perigraft soft-tissue attenuation, ectopic gas, pseudoaneurysm, or focal bowel wall thickening are applied.

▶ Indium-111 or technetium-99m hexametazime–labeled leukocytes is used as an adjunct to CT to identify graft infection.

▶ CT-guided aspiration can confirm infection and identify organism.

Management

▶ Graft replacement

▶ Antibiotics as an adjunct to surgery

Further Reading

Orton DF, LeVeen RF, Saigh JA, et al. Aortic prosthetic graft infections: radiologic manifestations and implications for management. *Radiographics*. 2000;20(4):977–993.

Section III   Adrenal

History

▶ 40-year-old man with incidental adrenal nodule

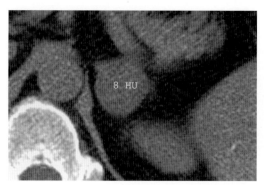

Figure 54.1

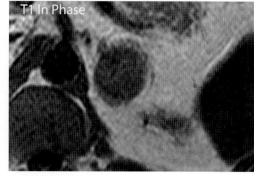

Figure 54.2

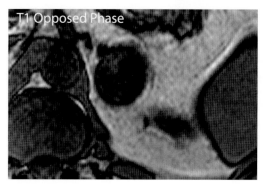

Figure 54.3

Case 54 Lipid-Rich Adrenal Adenoma

Findings

▶ Unenhanced CT imaging (Figure 54.1) shows a homogeneous low-attenuation adrenal nodule. The nodule is isointense on in-phase T1-weighted MR imaging (Figure 54.2) and shows prominent signal dropout on opposed-phase sequence (Figure 54.3).

Differential Diagnosis

▶ Homogeneous low attenuation (<10 HU) on CT and signal dropout on chemical shift oppose-phase imaging noted in this patient suggest the presence of microscopic fat, which is characteristic of lipid rich adrenal adenoma. Myelolipomas contain macroscopic fat, which is evident as large lipid-attenuation components on CT. They lose signal on fat-suppressed MR images but do not show signal loss on out-of-phase images. Metastases do not contain microscopic or macroscopic fat. Adrenal cortical carcinomas are aggressive, large, heterogeneous masses with necrosis.

Teaching Points

▶ Adrenal adenomas are present in 3% of autopsies.
▶ Presence of intracellular lipid is the most important diagnostic characteristic of adrenal adenoma.
▶ Seventy percent of adenomas are lipid rich and have substantial intracytoplasmic or microscopic fat, while the remainder are lipid poor.
▶ Lipid-rich adenomas have low attenuation on unenhanced CT. A threshold of 10 HU results in specificity of 98% and sensitivity of 71%.
▶ Chemical shift MR imaging identifies microscopic fat as signal loss on opposed-phase images.
▶ Chemical shift MR identifies adenomas with attenuation >10 HU on CT. Sensitivity of chemical shift MR for adenomas that measure between 10 and 30 HU is 89% but falls to 13% for adenomas that measure more than 30 HU.
▶ CT washout can diagnose lipid-poor adenomas in the absence of low-unenhanced attenuation.

Management

▶ Usually nonsurgical

Further Reading
Taffel M, Haji-Momenian S, Nikolaidis P, Miller FH. Adrenal imaging: a comprehensive review. *Radiol Clin North Am.* 2012;50(2):219–243.

History

▶ 50-year-old male with newly diagnosed lung cancer

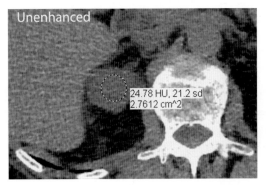

Figure 55.1

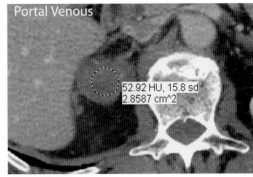

Figure 55.2

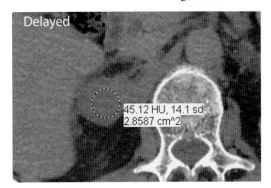

Figure 55.3

Case 55   Adrenal Metastasis

Findings

▶ CT adrenal washout study was performed. A right adrenal lesion enhances homogeneously on CT and has unenhanced attenuation of 24 HU (Figure 55.1), venous-phase attenuation of 52 HU (Figure 55.2), and 15-minute delay attenuation of 45 HU (Figure 55.3).

Differential Diagnosis

▶ The main diagnostic dilemma in a patient with primary malignancy and adrenal lesion is differentiating an incidental adenoma from metastasis. In this patient, the lesion does not contain microscopic fat identifiable by unenhanced CT. The absolute percentage washout calculated here is 45% {([enhanced HU − delayed HU]/ [enhanced HU − noncontrast HU]) × 100}. Absolute percentage washout <60% reflects slow washout and is concerning for malignancy. Pheochromocytoma and adrenal cortical cell carcinoma have similar washout characteristics. These are rare pathologies, and an adrenal metastasis from lung cancer is much more likely in this patient.

Teaching Points

▶ In the absence of a history of malignancy, likelihood of an adrenal mass being a metastasis is very low.
▶ Less than 0.2% of patients without known primary malignancy present with adrenal metastasis as the only manifestation of disease.
▶ In patients with known extra-adrenal malignancy, 50%–75% of adrenal masses represent metastases.
▶ Lung, breast, thyroid, and colon malignancies and melanoma are the most common source of adrenal metastases.
▶ Adrenal metastases tend to be large, less well defined, and heterogeneous on imaging.
▶ Metastases measure >10 HU on unenhanced CT and do not show signal loss on opposed-phase MRI.
▶ Metastases have slow contrast washout on delayed CT, with an absolute percentage washout of <60% at 15 minutes. This is due to delayed clearance of contrast by disorganized angiogenesis in metastases.
▶ Fludeoxyglucose positron emission tomography has a high sensitivity (91%) and specificity (97%) for adrenal metastases.

Management

▶ Varies with primary malignancy

Further Reading

Taffel M, Haji-Momenian S, Nikolaidis P, Miller FH. Adrenal imaging: a comprehensive review. *Radiol Clin North Am.* 2012;50(2):219–243.

Case 56

History

- 60-year-old man with recently diagnosed colon malignancy

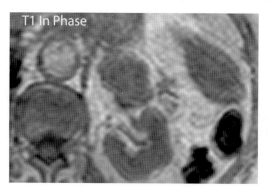

Figure 56.1

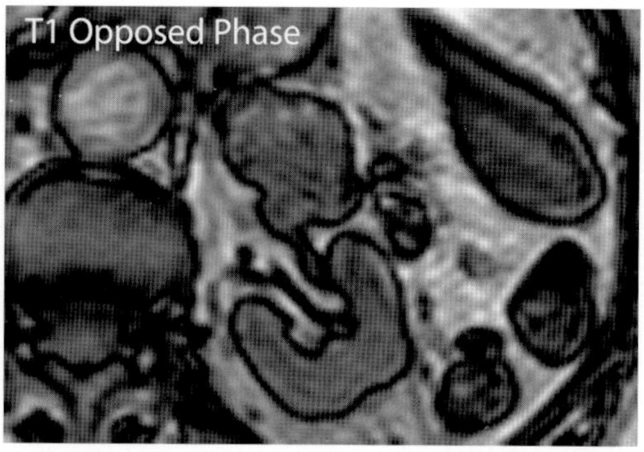

Figure 56.2

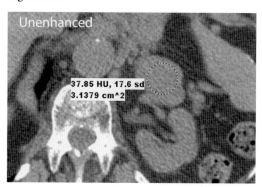

Figure 56.3

Figure 56.4

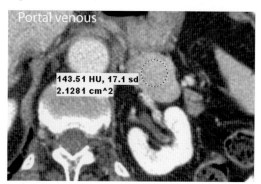

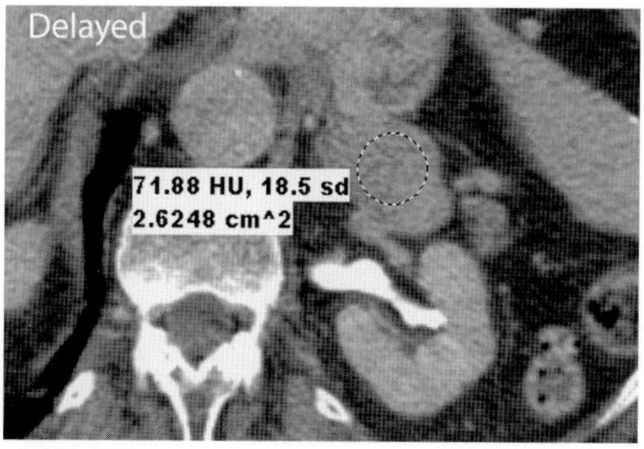

Figure 56.5

Case 56 Lipid-Poor Adrenal Adenoma

Findings

▶ T1-weighted in-phase (Figure 56.1) and opposed-phase (Figure 56.2) MR images show a T1 hypointense adrenal lesion that does not show signal drop on opposed-phase imaging.

▶ The lesion enhances homogeneously on CT and has unenhanced attenuation of 30 HU (Figure 56.3), venous-phase attenuation of 60 HU (Figure 56.4), and 15-minute delay attenuation of 45 HU (Figure 56.5).

Differential Diagnosis

▶ The main diagnostic dilemma in a patient with primary malignancy and adrenal lesion is differentiating an incidental adenoma from metastasis. In this patient, the lesion does not contain microscopic fat identifiable by unenhanced CT or chemical-shift MR, which excludes a lipid-rich adenoma. On adrenal washout study, the absolute percentage washout is 65% {([enhanced HU – delayed HU]/[enhanced HU – noncontrast HU]) × 100}. This is >60%, which excludes metastasis and confirms diagnosis of lipid-poor adrenal adenoma. Pheochromocytomas can occasionally mimic adenomas on washout studies but usually have a different clinical presentation.

Teaching Points

▶ Thirty percent of adrenal adenomas are lipid poor (unenhanced CT >10 HU).

▶ Lipid-poor and lipid-rich adenomas de-enhance faster after contrast administration compared with nonadenomatous lesions such as metastasis.

▶ Unenhanced 60-second and 15-minute delay CT images are used for washout calculation.

▶ Region of interest for attenuation measurement should cover half the lesion, avoiding cystic, necrotic, and calcified areas.

▶ An absolute percentage washout threshold of 60% results in 92% specificity and 86% sensitivity for lipid-poor adenomas.

▶ If unenhanced CT is not available, then relative percentage washout can be calculated from the portal venous and delayed attenuations using the following formula: ([enhanced HU – delayed HU]/enhanced HU) × 100.

▶ Relative washout threshold of 40% results in 92% specificity and 82% sensitivity for lipid-poor adenomas.

Management

▶ Nonsurgical

Further Reading

Taffel M, Haji-Momenian S, Nikolaidis P, Miller FH. Adrenal imaging: a comprehensive review. *Radiol Clin North Am.* 2012;50(2):219–243.

History

▶ 35-year-old female with acute elevation of blood pressure

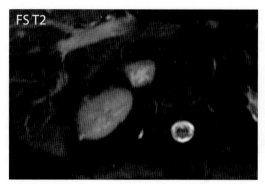

Figure 57.1

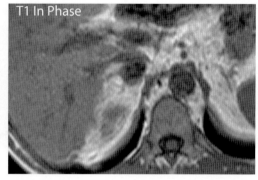

Figure 57.2

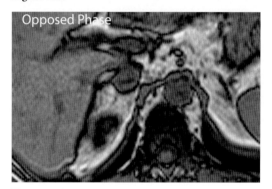

Figure 57.3

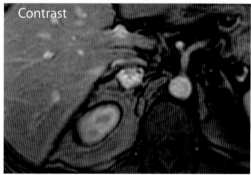

Figure 57.4

Case 57 Pheochromocytoma

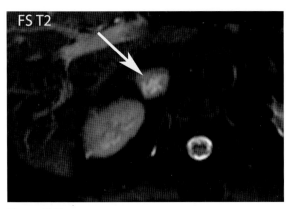

Figure 57.5

Findings

▶ MRI images show a well-defined right adrenal lesion that is markedly hyperintense on the fat-suppressed T2-weighted images (Figure 57.1; arrow in Figure 57.5). It is predominantly isointense with some hypointense areas on in-phase T1-weighted images (Figure 57.2) and does not show signal loss on opposed-phase images (Figure 57.3). It shows intense contrast enhancement (Figure 57.4).

Differential Diagnosis

▶ Lipid-rich adrenal adenomas show signal dropout on opposed-phase imaging, myelolipomas lose signal on fat-suppressed sequences, and adrenal hemorrhage is hyperintense on T1 imaging. Lipid-poor adenomas and metastases do not have specific imaging features on MRI but are usually iso- to mildly hyperintense on T2 and show mild to moderate enhancement. High T2 signal intensity, absence of micro- or macroscopic fat, and intense enhancement are suggestive of adrenal pheochromocytoma in a patient presenting with hypertensive crisis.

Teaching Points

▶ Pheochromocytomas are catecholamine-secreting tumors; 90% arise from chromaffin cells in adrenal medulla.
▶ Catecholamine release causes paroxysmal episodes that are associated with hypertension, palpitations, and diaphoresis.
▶ The 10% rule applies, that is, 10% pheochromocytomas are extra-adrenal, 10% are bilateral (usually syndromic), 10% occur in children, 10% are nonfunctioning, and 10% are malignant.
▶ They are associated with multiple endocrine neoplasia, type II ; von Hippel–Lindau syndrome; and neurofibromatosis.
▶ Most common imaging appearance is high T2 signal intensity, low T1 signal intensity, and avid enhancement.
▶ Imaging features are variable, and up to 35% pheochromocytomas have low T2 signal.
▶ Pheochromocytomas are usually solid but can be cystic or contain calcium, hemorrhage, and fat.
▶ Metaiodobenzylguanidine and octreotide scanning have high specificity but low sensitivity for pheochromocytoma.
▶ Urinary and plasma catecholamine levels have high sensitivity for pheochromocytoma.
▶ Biopsy is contraindicated and may precipitate hypertensive crisis.

Management

▶ Surgery

Further Reading

Colby GW, Banks KP, Torres E. AJR teaching file: incidental adrenal mass and hypertension. *AJR Am J Roentgenol.* 2006;187(3 suppl):S470–472.

History

▶ 40-year-old woman with lower extremity edema

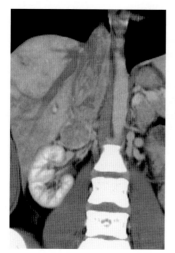

Figure 58.1

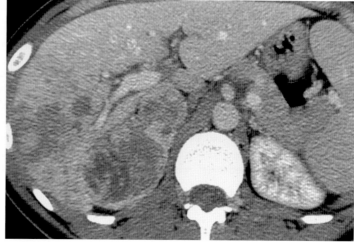

Figure 58.2

Case 58 Adrenal Cortical Carcinoma

Findings

▶ Contrast-enhanced CT images show a large, heterogeneously enhancing mass involving the right adrenal gland (Figures 58.1 and 58.2). Tumor extends into the suprahepatic inferior vena cava (IVC). Heterogeneous enhancement of the liver is secondary to thrombus in the right hepatic vein.

Differential Diagnosis

▶ The heterogeneous enhancement, large size, and IVC invasion establish the malignant nature of the mass. Although metastases are the most common malignant adrenal pathology, they are unusual in the absence of a known primary malignancy. Direct IVC invasion by an adrenal metastasis is also highly unlikely. IVC invasion is a typical feature of adrenal cortical carcinoma (ACC). The large size and heterogeneous enhancement noted here are compatible with ACC. IVC invasion is seen in renal cell and hepatocellular carcinoma, but the organ of origin is usually obvious in these patients. Pheochromocytomas have varied imaging appearances and can be malignant, but IVC invasion is not a feature of pheochromocytoma. Adrenal adenomas are benign, small, homogeneous lesions and therefore excluded. ACC is the favored diagnosis here.

Teaching Points

▶ ACCs are rare aggressive tumors with incidence of 1–2 per million per year.

▶ They show bimodal age distribution, with peaks in the first and fourth/fifth decades.

▶ Mean size at presentation is 10 cm.

▶ Fifteen to thirty percent of ACCs are functional in adults (more common in children).

▶ Functional tumors present with Cushing syndrome, virilization, or feminization.

▶ Nonfunctioning tumors present due to mass effect; 30% of ACCs are metastatic at presentation.

▶ Features that suggest diagnosis of ACC include size >4 cm, irregular margins, necrosis, hemorrhage, calcification, heterogeneous enhancement, and invasion of IVC/renal vein or adjacent structure.

▶ ACCs do not preferentially washout on delayed images.

▶ It can be difficult to differentiate adenoma from ACC on biopsy specimens.

▶ Indeterminate adrenal lesions >4 cm are treated as malignant lesions.

Management

▶ Surgical excision; recurrence and metastases are common

Further Reading

Bharwani N, Rockall AG, Sahdev A, et al. Adrenocortical carcinoma: the range of appearances on CT and MRI. *AJR Am J Roentgenol.* 2011;196(6):W706–714.

History

► Motor vehicle accident; CT images on admission (Figure 59.1) and follow-up at 24 hours
(Figure 59.2) and 2 weeks (Figure 59.3) are provided

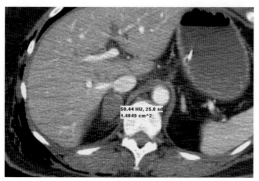

Figure 59.1

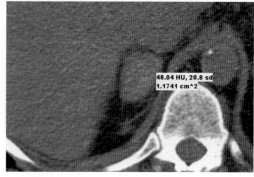

Figure 59.2

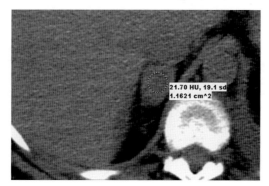

Figure 59.3

Case 59   Adrenal Hemorrhage

Findings

▶ Contrast-enhanced CT image (Figure 59.1) shows a high-attenuation (50 HU), ovoid, right adrenal nodule (region-of-interest circle) with adjacent fat stranding. Right flank subcutaneous emphysema is present.

▶ Follow-up unenhanced CT (Figure 59.2) after 24 hours shows high attenuation (48 HU) of adrenal nodule.

▶ Repeat unenhanced CT after 2 weeks (Figure 59.3) shows decrease in size and attenuation (21 HU) of adrenal nodule.

Differential Diagnosis

▶ The diagnostic dilemma with this contrast-enhanced trauma CT is determining whether the high attenuation of the adrenal nodule is due to traumatic adrenal hemorrhage or represents enhancement in an incidental adenoma (by far, the most common adrenal lesion). Presence of adjacent flank emphysema indicates significant trauma, which is a common setting for adrenal hemorrhage. Periadrenal stranding and ovoid shape also favor adrenal hematoma. The diagnosis is confirmed on follow-up unenhanced CT after 24 hours; the image shows high attenuation, which is consistent with hemorrhage. Adenomas have low attenuation on unenhanced CT. Repeat CT obtained after 2 weeks demonstrates interval decrease in attenuation and size, typical of an evolving hematoma.

Teaching Points

▶ Trauma is the most common cause of adrenal hemorrhage.

▶ Nontraumatic causes of adrenal hemorrhage include stress due to surgery, infection or burns, coagulopathy, and tumor.

▶ Adrenal hemorrhage is seen in 2% of patients undergoing abdominal CT for trauma.

▶ Traumatic adrenal hemorrhage is usually unilateral (95%) and more common on the right side (77%).

▶ It is associated with other substantial visceral, chest, or orthopedic injury in the vast majority of patients. Careful search for other injury is warranted.

▶ Acute primary adrenal insufficiency (Addisonian crisis) occurs only when hemorrhage destroys 90% of both glands. Nontraumatic bilateral adrenal hemorrhage is usually seen secondary to stress or coagulopathy.

▶ Mean attenuation of acute adrenal hemorrhage is 52 HU and generally 40–60 HU.

Management

▶ Conservative

Further Reading
Rana AI, Kenney PJ, Lockhart ME, et al. Adrenal gland hematomas in trauma patients. *Radiology*. 2004;230(3):669–675.

History

▶ 35-year-old female with incidental adrenal lesion

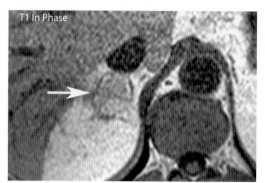

Figure 60.1

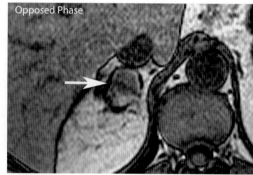

Figure 60.2

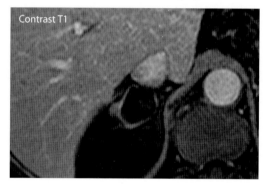

Figure 60.3

Case 60   Adrenal Myelolipoma

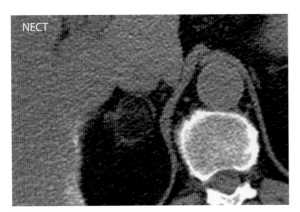

Figure 60.4

Findings

▶ A well-defined right adrenal nodule is present that is hyperintense on T1-weighted in-phase image (arrow in Figure 60.1) and does not show signal drop on opposed-phase image (arrow in Figure 60.2). The lesion is predominantly hypointense and nonenhancing on the fat-suppressed contrast-enhanced T1-weighted image (Figure 60.3).

▶ The lesion is predominantly lipid attenuation on unenhanced CT with wisps of higher-attenuation tissue (Figure 60.4).

Differential Diagnosis

▶ On in-phase T1-weighted image, the adrenal nodule has high signal similar to retroperitoneal fat and does not significantly change on opposed-phase imaging. The nodule follows signal intensity of adjacent retroperitoneal fat and becomes hypointense on the fat-suppressed contrast-enhanced T1-weighted image. This confirms macroscopic fat within the nodule and is diagnostic of myelolipoma. Adrenal adenomas contain microscopic fat. Microscopic fat loses signal on opposed-phase imaging but not on fat-suppressed T1-weighted imaging.

Teaching Points

▶ Adrenal myelolipomas are benign tumors that contain mature fat interspersed with hematopoietic elements.
▶ Myelolipomas are usually asymptomatic and, rarely, can present with hemorrhage.
▶ Myelolipomas have macroscopic fat on imaging.
▶ A variable amount of macroscopic fat with negative attenuation value (generally <-20 HU) is interspersed between higher-attenuation elements.
▶ High T1 signal and suppression on fat-suppressed sequences identify macroscopic fat on magnetic resonance imaging.
▶ Myelolipomas show T2 hyperintensity due to presence of marrow-like elements.
▶ Myelolipomas are predominantly hyperechoic on ultrasound.
▶ Rarely, myelolipomas can coexist with another adrenal lesion such as adenoma. The imaging findings are not typical of either lesion in these cases.

Management

▶ No follow-up or intervention is required, unless there is symptomatic hemorrhage.

Further Reading

Rao P, Kenney PJ, Wagner BJ, Davidson AJ. Imaging and pathologic features of myelolipoma. *Radiographics.* 1997;17(6):1373–1385.

History

▶ 25-year-old following motor vehicle accident

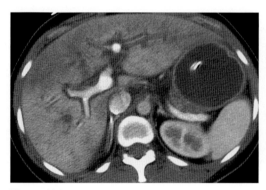

Figure 61.1

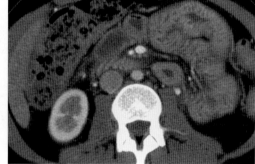

Figure 61.2

61 Intense Adrenal Enhancement in Hypoperfusion Complex (Shock Adrenals)

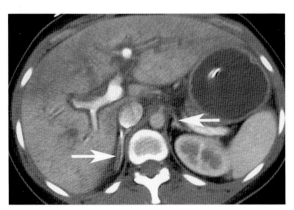

Figure 61.3

Findings

▶ Contrast-enhanced CT images (Figures 61.1 and 61.2) show intense enhancement of otherwise normal-appearing adrenals (arrow in Figure 61.3). Heterogeneous enhancement of the liver, small bowel mucosal enhancement, and a small caliber aorta are noted.

Differential Diagnosis

▶ The maintenance of normal adreniform shape without focal nodule and intense enhancement (equal to or more than adjacent vascular structures) of both glands is pathognomic of hypoperfusion complex and is known as shock adrenals. The liver, small bowel, and aorta findings also support the diagnosis in this case. Adrenal hemorrhage typically is associated with focal enlargement and has lower density.

Teaching Points

▶ Hypoperfusion complex refers to a combination of findings on CT, most commonly seen in patients with significant blood loss after severe trauma.
▶ Etiology of intense adrenal enhancement is not known but likely related to sympathetic response to hypovolemic shock.
▶ Adrenal hyperenhancement is also seen in conditions other than hypovolemic shock such as severe burns, severe acute pancreatitis, and cardiac arrest.
▶ Other manifestations of hypoperfusion complex include small caliber aorta, flattening of inferior vena cava, heterogeneous hepatic enhancement, peripancreatic edema and abnormal pancreatic enhancement, splenic hypoperfusion, intense prolonged renal enhancement, and increased small bowel mucosal enhancement.
▶ Intense adrenal enhancement has been suggested to be a poor prognostic marker in trauma patients.

Management

▶ Supportive management is recommended. Intense enhancement in normal-shaped adrenals can be an early marker for impending shock.

Further Reading

O'Hara SM, Donnelly LF. Intense contrast enhancement of the adrenal glands: another abdominal CT finding associated with hypoperfusion complex in children. *AJR Am J Roentgenol*. 1999;173(4):995–997.

History

▶ 48-year-old woman with weight gain and fatigue; laboratory results reveal suppressed adrenocorticotropic hormone (ACTH) level and increased cortisol

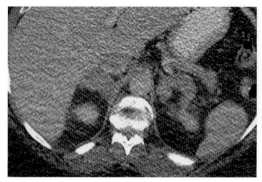

Figure 62.1

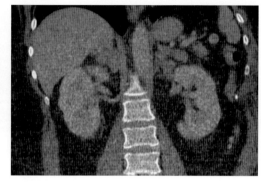

Figure 62.2

Case 62   Adrenal Hyperplasia

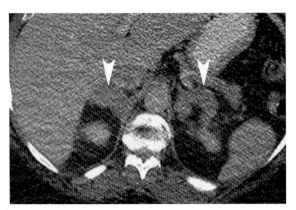

Figure 62.3

Findings

▶ Contrast-enhanced CT images (Figures 62.1 and 62.2) show massive nodular enlargement of bilateral adrenal glands with maintenance of the adreniform shape (arrowheads in Figure 62.3).

Differential Diagnosis

▶ In the absence of exogenous steroid administration, suppressed ACTH level with elevated cortisol suggests ACTH-independent Cushing syndrome. Adrenal adenomas are the most common cause of ACTH-independent Cushing syndrome. However, no focal adenoma is identified here. Bilateral adrenal enlargement with maintenance of adrenaliform shape, as noted here, is more consistent with diffuse adrenal hyperplasia. ACTH-independent macronodular adrenocortical hyperplasia is characterized by bilateral massive nodular and is the favored diagnosis. Primary pigmented adrenal nodular disease also causes diffuse adrenal hyperplasia and ACTH-independent hypercortisolism but is characterized by small bilateral nodules and is less likely.

Teaching Points

▶ Functional clinical syndromes associated with adrenocortical hyperplasia include ACTH-dependent or -independent Cushing syndrome, primary aldosteronism, and congenital adrenal hyperplasia.

▶ Endogenous Cushing syndrome (hypercortisolism) is ACTH dependent (80%–85%) or less commonly ACTH independent (15%–20%).

▶ Seventy percent of patients with ACTH-dependent hypercortisolism have diffuse or nodular thickening of the adrenals.

▶ The vast majority (95%) of ACTH-independent hypercortisolism is due to adrenal adenoma or adrenocortical carcinoma.

▶ Bilateral adrenal hyperplasia is responsible for the other types of ACTH-independent hypercortisolism (5%). Most of these are due to primary pigmented adrenal nodular disease and the minority are due ACTH-independent macronodular adrenocortical hyperplasia.

▶ Primary hyperaldosteronism is caused by either bilateral adrenal hyperplasia or adenoma.

▶ In a large percentage, adrenocortical hyperplasia is a radiographic finding of unknown cause without clinical or biochemical manifestations.

▶ Average width of each adrenal limb in the normal population is 3 mm; a thickness of 5 mm is considered enlarged. The adrenal body is enlarged if the width is >1 cm on the right and >1.2 cm on the left.

Management

▶ Adrenalectomy often done for Cushing syndrome

Further Reading

Schteingart DE. The clinical spectrum of adrenocortical hyperplasia. *Curr Opin Endocrinol Diabetes Obes.* 2012;19(3):176–182.

History

▶ 50-year-old man with lung cancer with adrenal mass

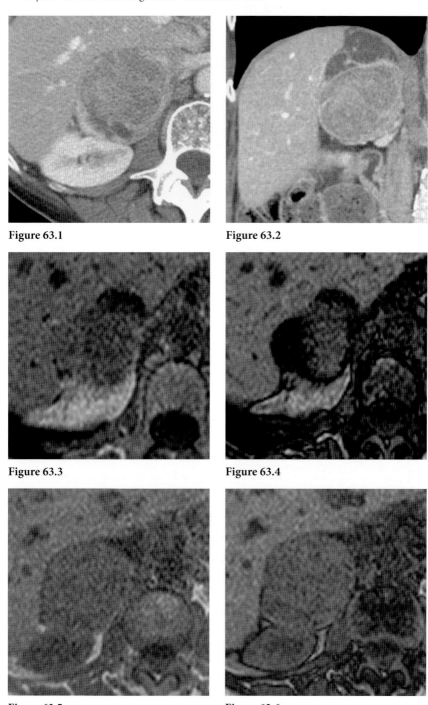

Figure 63.1

Figure 63.2

Figure 63.3

Figure 63.4

Figure 63.5

Figure 63.6

Case 63   Adrenal Collision Tumor

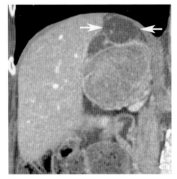
Figure 63.7

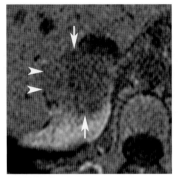
Figure 63.8

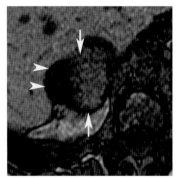
Figure 63.9

Findings

▶ Contrast-enhanced CT images (Figures 63.1 and 63.2) show a heterogeneously enhancing right adrenal mass. The cranial part of the tumor (arrows in Figure 63.7) is more homogeneous and lower attenuation than the larger, heterogeneous caudal component.

▶ T1-weighted in-phase and corresponding opposed-phase images through cranial part of lesion (Figures 63.3 and 63.4) show loss of signal on opposed-phase imaging in the lateral component of the lesion (arrowheads in Figures 63.8 and 63.9). Medial component does not show signal loss (arrows in Figures 63.8 and 63.9).

▶ In-phase and opposed-phase images through the caudal part of the lesion (Figures 63.5 and 63.6) do not demonstrate any signal loss on the opposed-phase sequence.

Differential Diagnosis

▶ In a patient with known primary malignancy, the main differential of an adrenal mass is metastasis versus adenoma. Adrenal adenomas are usually homogeneous and contain microscopic fat. Microscopic fat results in lower CT attenuation and signal loss on opposed-phase MRI. Adrenal metastases are heterogeneous and do not contain microscopic fat. In this patient, features of both adenoma and metastasis are present in adjacent parts of the lesion. The cranial part is homogeneous, low attenuation on CT, and shows signal loss on opposed-phase MRI (consistent with microscopic fat), typical of an adenoma. The caudal part is heterogeneous without signal loss on opposed-phase imaging, consistent with metastasis. This is suggestive of an adrenal collision tumor comprising adenoma and metastasis.

Teaching Points

▶ Collision tumors represent coexistence of two adjacent but histologically distinct tumors without admixture.

▶ Collision tumors can constitute two malignant tumors (lymphoma and adenocarcinoma) or a benign and a malignant tumor (adenoma and metastasis).

▶ Adenomas and metastases are both common adrenal lesions. Subsequent metastasis to an adrenal with a preexisting adenoma will lead to formation of an adrenal collision tumor.

Management

▶ Resection

Further Reading
Schwartz LH, Macari M, Huvos AG, Panicek DM. Collision tumors of the adrenal gland: demonstration and characterization at MR imaging. *Radiology.* 1996;201(3):757–260.

History

▶ 36-year-old woman with incidental left adrenal lesion

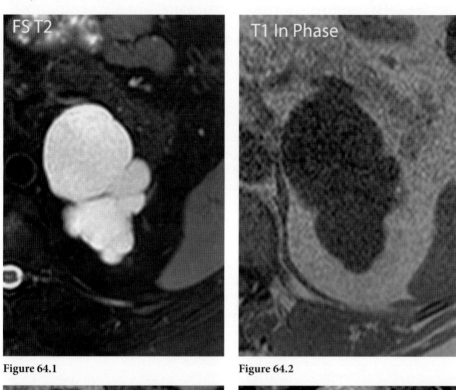

Figure 64.1

Figure 64.2

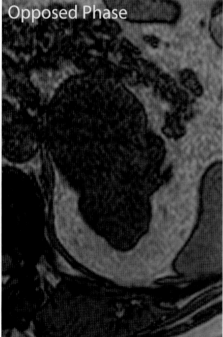

Figure 64.3

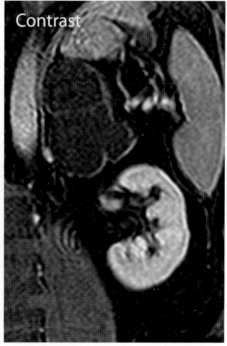

Figure 64.4

Case 64 Adrenal Endothelial Cyst (Lymphangioma)

Findings

▶ Fat-suppressed T2-weighted MR image (Figure 64.1) shows a T2 hyperintense multiloculated cyst with thin septations. The cyst is hypointense on in-phase T1-weighted image (Figure 64.2) and does not show any change on opposed-phase image (Figure 64.3). Coronal contrast-enhanced fat-suppressed T1-weighted image (Figure 64.4) shows mild, smooth enhancement of the cyst wall.

Differential Diagnosis

▶ Differential diagnosis of cystic adrenal lesions includes endothelial cysts (commonly lymphangiomas), pseudocysts, and occasionally malignant tumors with cystic change. Absence of any nodularity or significant wall thickening excludes a malignant etiology. It is difficult to differentiate between common benign cystic adrenal lesions on imaging due to overlapping features. Lymphangiomas are more frequently multilocular than pseudocysts, while pseudocysts often contain blood products. Multilocularity and absence of blood products on MRI slightly favor the diagnosis of lymphangioma in this case.

Teaching Points

▶ Adrenal cysts are rare, with a prevalence of 0.06%–0.18%.
▶ Adrenal cysts are usually asymptomatic.
▶ Most adrenal cysts are benign. Histologically 45% are endothelial cysts, 39% are pseudocysts, and 9% are epithelial cysts.
▶ Ninety-three percent of endothelial cysts are lymphangiomas and the rest are hemangiomas.
▶ Occasionally other adrenal tumors such as pheochromocytoma and adrenal cortical cell carcinoma undergo cystic degeneration.
▶ Hemorrhage is often present in andrenal pseudocyst and may be the underlying cause for cyst formation.
▶ More than 50% of adrenal cysts (endothelial and pseudocysts) have wall calcification.
▶ Most benign adrenal cysts have mild wall thickening (2–3 mm). Unlike renal cysts, mild wall thickening is not considered a worrisome feature.

Management

▶ Observation or surgical excision

Further Reading
Rozenblit A, Morehouse HT, Amis ES Jr. Cystic adrenal lesions: CT features. *Radiology*. 1996;201(2):541–548.

Section IV Ureter and Bladder

History

▶ 70-year-old male with hematuria

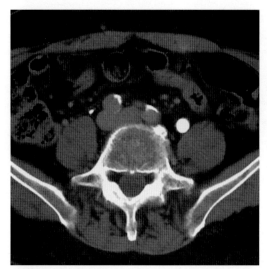

Figure 65.1

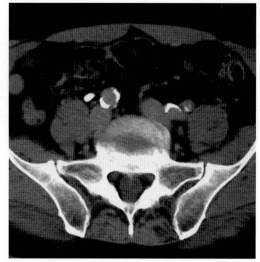

Figure 65.2

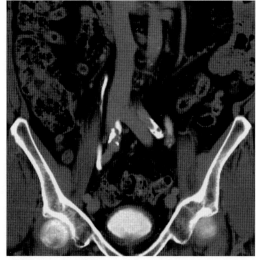

Figure 65.3

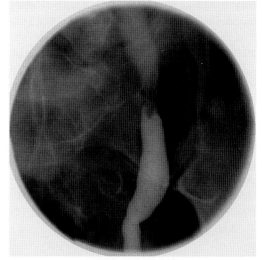

Figure 65.4

Case 65 Ureteric Transitional Cell Carcinoma

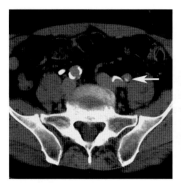 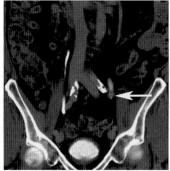 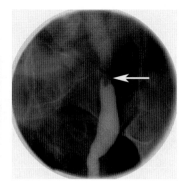

Figure 65.5   **Figure 65.6**   **Figure 65.7**

Findings

▶ Axial excretory-phase image (Figure 65.1) shows a dilated left ureter. A more distal axial image (Figure 65.2) shows a soft tissue nodule occluding the left ureter (arrow in Figure 65.5). A coronal image (Figure 65.3) also demonstrates the left ureteral mass (arrow in Figure 65.6).

▶ Retrograde ureterogram (Figure 65.4) demonstrates a filling defect occluding the left ureter (arrow in Figure 65.7).

Differential Diagnosis

▶ Ureteric calculus is the most common cause of ureteric obstruction and can be easily identified on CT images. Benign ureteral strictures cause gradual tapering of the ureter without any associated soft tissue. A focal-enhancing soft-tissue attenuation-filling defect in the ureter, as noted here, is most concerning for urothelial malignancy. In this patient, urothelial malignancy was confirmed on ureteroscopic biopsy.

Teaching Points

▶ Transitional cell carcinoma (TCC) is the most common urothelial malignancy.

▶ Bladder is the most common site of TCC, with only 5% of cases involving the collecting system and ureters.

▶ TCC is often multifocal; approximately 30%–50% of patients with upper tract TCC develop bladder TCC.

▶ There is a male preponderance, with a peak incidence in the seventh decade.

▶ Hematuria is a common presentation.

▶ Opacification of the collecting system and ureters during excretory-phase imaging in CT urogram helps identify urothelial malignancy as small soft tissue filling defects.

▶ Unlike bladder TCCs, the majority of upper tract TCCs are invasive.

▶ The diagnosis is usually confirmed by biopsy during retrograde ureteroscopy.

Management

▶ Due to the potential for multifocal tumors, nephroureterectomy is usually performed for upper tract TCC.

Further Reading
Vikram R, Sandler CM, Ng CS. Imaging and staging of transitional cell carcinoma: part 2, upper urinary tract. *AJR Am J Roentgenol.* 2009;192(6):1488–1493.

History

▶ 55-year-old female with previous cystectomy and acute renal failure underwent a conduitogram (Figure 66.1) and subsequent anterograde nephrostogram (Figure 66.2)

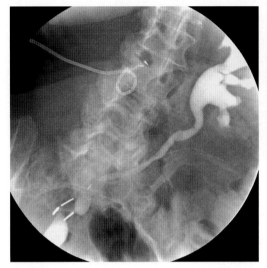

Figure 66.1

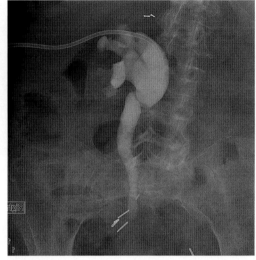

Figure 66.2

Case 66   Conduit Stenosis

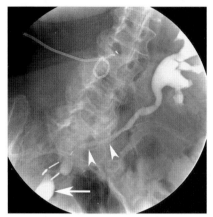
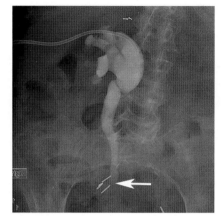

Figure 66.3   **Figure 66.4**

Findings

▶ Ileal conduitogram (Figure 66.1) shows opacification of the ileal conduit (arrow in Figure 66.3) with reflux of contrast into the left ureter (arrowheads) and collecting system. There is no reflux of contrast into the right ureter. A right nephrostomy catheter is noted.

▶ Right antegrade nephrostogram (Figure 66.2) through nephrostomy tube shows severe dilation of the right collecting system and ureter. Abrupt distal right ureteric narrowing is present (arrow in Figure 66.4). Contrast does not opacify the ileal conduit.

Differential Diagnosis

▶ Post-cystectomy patients with ureteric implantation into an ileal conduit are susceptible to development of stenosis at the ureteroenterostomy. In this patient, reflux of contrast into the left ureter during the conduitogram suggests patency of the left ureteroenteric anastomosis. Absence of reflux into the right ureter during the conduitogram could be due to stenosis at the right ureteroenteric anastomosis, antirefluxing surgical technique, distal ureteric recurrence of primary neoplasm, or underdistention of the conduit. The antegrade nephrostogram confirms a right distal ureteric/ureteroenteric anastomotic stenosis. Pouchoscopy confirmed severe stenosis at the right ureteroenteric anastomosis.

Teaching Points

▶ Bladder malignancies are commonly treated with cystectomy and neobladder formation using an ileal conduit.

▶ Conduitograms are performed by retrograde administration of contrast into a neobladder after urinary diversion surgery to evaluate the conduit and the upper tracts.

▶ Ileal conduits are susceptible to obstruction, reflux, and infection.

▶ Stenosis at the ureteroenteric anastomosis is a complication of urinary diversion and usually occurs within 2 years of surgery.

▶ Distal ureteric obstruction can also be secondary to recurrence of urothelial neoplasm.

Management

▶ Surgical revision, balloon dilation, or stenting

Further Reading

Hautmann RE. Urinary diversion: ileal conduit to neobladder. *J Urol.* 2003;169(3):834–842.

History

▶ 52-year-old man with severe acute left flank pain

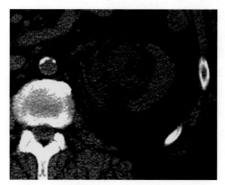

Figures 67.1

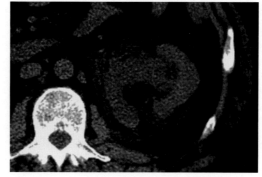

Figures 67.2

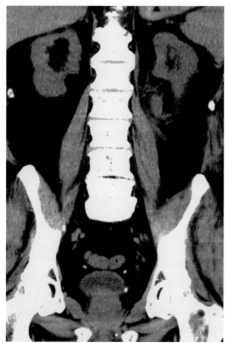

Figures 67.3

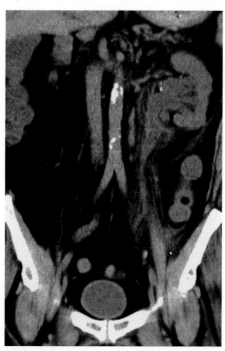

Figures 67.4

Case 67   Ureteral Calculus with Pyelocalyceal Rupture

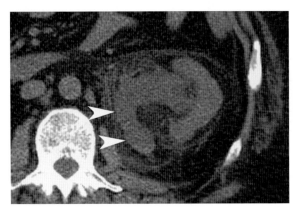

Figures 67.5   **Figures 67.6**

Findings

▶ Unenhanced axial and coronal CT images (Figures 67.1–67.4) show left hydroureteronephrosis with extensive stranding around the left renal pelvis and ureter. A urine leak into the perinephric space from the left renal pelvis is present (arrowheads in Figure 67.5). An obstructing left ureterovesical junction calculus is noted (arrow in Figure 67.6).

Differential Diagnosis

▶ Common causes of perinephric fluid include trauma, surgical intervention, and infection. No history of trauma or surgical intervention is present in this patient. Lack of fever, leukocytosis, and other systemic manifestations of sepsis make infection with perinephric abscess formation unlikely. Pyelocalyceal/fornicial rupture secondary to increased pyelocalyceal pressure in an obstructed system is an unusual cause of perinephric fluid. Left hydroureteronephrosis and perinephric/periureteric stranding, as noted here, are consistent with acute ureteral obstruction. Demonstration of the left ureterovesical junction calculus confirms the diagnosis of pyelocalyceal rupture secondary to obstructive urolithiasis. Tumor can also cause ureteral obstruction and needs to be excluded.

Teaching Points

▶ Urolithiasis is commonly seen in those aged 30–60 years, with a male preponderance.
▶ Diet, genetics, geography, and urinary tract infections are among various factors associated with urolithiasis.
▶ Hypercalciuria and hyperuricosuria due to any cause can cause urolithiasis.
▶ Urinary stones have varied composition, with calcium-containing stone (including oxalate and phosphate) comprising 70%–80%, mixed struvite and apatite 15%, uric acid 8%, and cystine 3%.
▶ Uric acid stones can be treated by urine alkalinization. Urine pH, urinary crystals, and presence of urease-splitting organisms are used to identify uric acid calculi.

Management

▶ Ureteral stones 5 mm or smaller pass spontaneously in 68% of patients and stones 6–10 mm in size pass spontaneously in 47% of patients. Larger stones or stones refractory to medical therapy are removed by extracorporeal shockwave lithotripsy, ureteroscopy, or percutaneous nephrolithotomy.

Further Reading

Kambadakone AR, Eisner BH, Catalano OA, Sahani DV. New and evolving concepts in the imaging and management of urolithiasis: urologists' perspective. *Radiographics*. 2010;30(3):603–623.

Case 68

History

► 55-year-old female with microhematuria

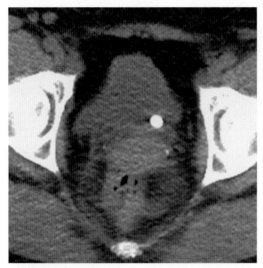

Figure 68.1

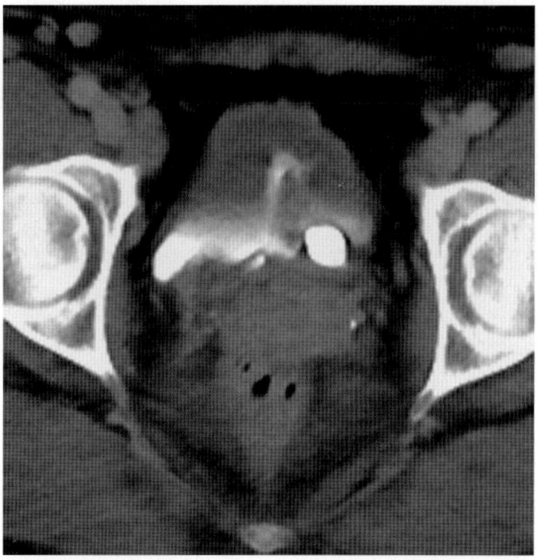

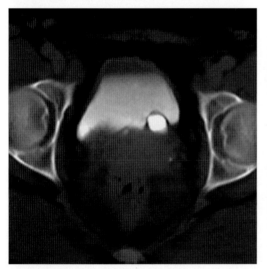

Figure 68.2

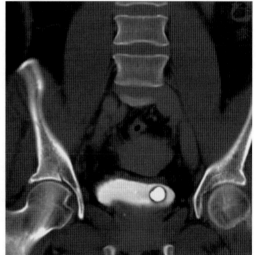

Figure 68.3

Figure 68.4

Case 68   Ureterocele

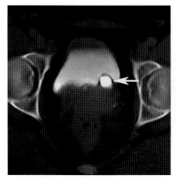
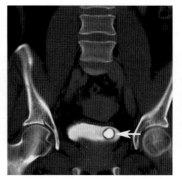
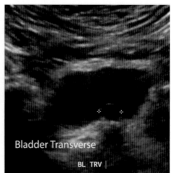

Figure 68.5   **Figure 68.6**   **Figure 68.7**

Findings

▶ Unenhanced CT image (Figure 68.1) of the pelvis shows a large calcification in the region of the left ureteric orifice.
▶ Post-contrast–delayed images (Figures 68.2–68.4) show the calcification to be within a contrast-filled outpouching at the ureteric orifice, which extends medially and protrudes into the bladder. Arrows in Figures 68.5 and 68.6 and point to the low-attenuation thin rim of ureteric tissue, which helps identify this calculus/urine-filled sac.
▶ Pelvic ultrasound image from a different patient (Figure 68.7) shows a thin-walled sac protruding into the bladder at the ureteric orifice (calipers).

Differential Diagnosis

▶ On the CT images, the contrast-filled outpouching at the ureteric orifice, as noted here, is characteristic of a ureterocele. Urinary stasis can result in development of calculi within a ureterocele. Impacted stone and bladder tumor, which can mimic this appearance, have been described as causes of pseudoureteroceles on intravenous urograms. Demonstration of a rim of ureteric tissue helps differentiate ureteroceles from calculi impacted at the ureterovesicle junction. Tumors are identified as soft tissue masses.
▶ On ultrasound, ureteroceles typically appear as thin-walled cystic structures that protrude into the bladder lumen at the ureteric orifice, as seen in Figure 68.7.

Teaching Points

▶ Ureteroceles arise due to congenital weakness of the bladder wall at the ureteric orifice.
▶ Ureteroceles can be unilateral or bilateral.
▶ Most ureteroceles are asymptomatic.
▶ Ureteric obstruction by large ureteroceles, calculi formation due to stasis, and infection can cause symptoms.
▶ Ectopic ureteroceles occur when there is ectopic insertion of the ureter. They are always associated with duplication of the ureter and arise from the ureter draining the upper pole moiety (Weigart–Meyer rule).
▶ On intravenous urograms, ureteroceles are identified by dilation of the distal end of the ureter with a thin surrounding radiolucent halo. This is known as the "cobra head" or "spring onion" sign.

Management

▶ Treatment is reserved for symptomatic cases.

Further Reading
Chavhan GB. The cobra head sign. *Radiology*. 2002;*225*(3):781–782.

History

▶ 72-year-old man with hematuria

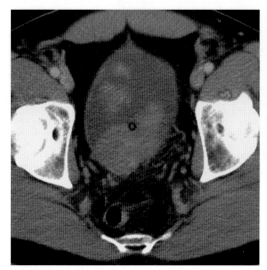

Figure 69.1

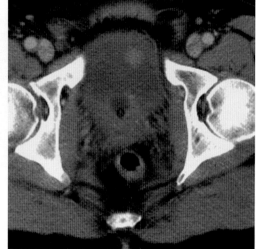

Figure 69.2

Case 69 Bladder Cancer

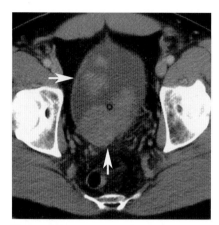

Figure 69.3

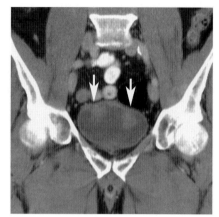

Figure 69.4

Findings

▶ Axial and coronal contrast-enhanced CT images (Figures 69.1 and 69.2) show multiple enhancing polypoid bladder wall masses (arrows in Figures 69.3 and 69.4).

Differential Diagnosis

▶ Differential diagnosis of soft-tissue attenuation lesions in the bladder includes urothelial carcinoma and blood clot. Blood clots are usually in the dependent part of the bladder and do not enhance. In this patient, the enhancement and nondependent position of the nodules are consistent with multifocal urothelial malignancy.

Teaching Points

▶ Transitional cell carcinoma constitutes 95% of urothelial malignancies, the majority of the remainder being squamous cell carcinoma.

▶ Painless hematuria is the most frequent clinical presentation.

▶ Transitional cell carcinoma occurs in older patients (median age 69 years), with male preponderance.

▶ Cystoscopy is used for diagnosis and local staging of bladder carcinoma. CT does not identify bladder wall invasion, and small tumors may not be visible on CT due to inadequate distention.

▶ Bladder tumors without muscle invasion have very low risk of metastases and are resected without any further disease staging.

▶ Muscle-invasive tumors are at higher risk of metastases and undergo CT for staging.

▶ Curative surgery or radiotherapy is attempted only in patients without nodal disease.

▶ Obturator, presacral, and internal and external iliac nodes are considered regional nodes, while common iliac involvement is considered distant metastasis.

▶ Presence of lymph nodal metastases adversely affects the outcome such that the 3-year survival is 70% without lymph nodal metastasis, 50% with one lymph node involvement, and 25% with multiple lymph node involvement.

Management

▶ Cystoscopic excision for early disease; chemotherapy, radiation, and surgery for more advanced disease

Further Reading

Purysko AS, Leão Filho HM, Herts BR. Radiologic imaging of patients with bladder cancer. *Semin Oncol.* 2012;39(5):543–548.

History

▶ 66-year-old male with hematuria

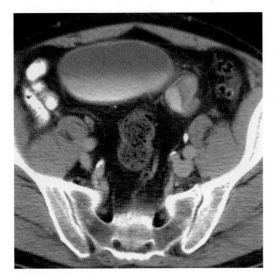

Figure 70.1

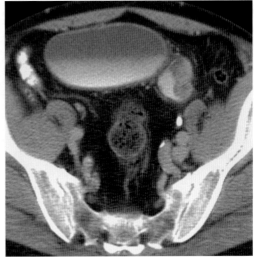

Figure 70.2

Case 70 Bladder Cancer Within a Diverticulum

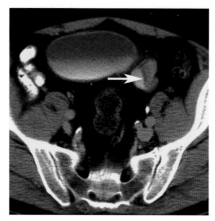

Figure 70.3

Findings

▶ Contrast-enhanced CT images (Figures 70.1 and 70.2) show a focal left lateral bladder wall diverticulum. Nodular-enhancing soft-tissue attenuation is noted within the diverticulum (arrow in Figure 70.3).

Differential Diagnosis

▶ Differential diagnosis of a focal lesion in a bladder diverticulum includes stone, blood clot, and urothelial carcinoma. Bladder stones are usually calcified and can be excluded. Blood clots do not enhance and are located in the dependent part of the bladder. In this patient, the enhancing nodule along the lateral aspect of the bladder diverticulum is consistent with urothelial malignancy arising in a diverticulum.

Teaching Points

▶ Bladder diverticula lack a muscular layer as they are caused by herniation of bladder mucosa through areas of weakness in the detrusor muscle.
▶ Urinary stasis in diverticula results in chronic infection and inflammation.
▶ Transitional cell carcinoma (TCC) is the most common tumor in a bladder diverticulum.
▶ Due to the lack of a muscular layer, which serves as a barrier to tumor spread, tumors in bladder diverticula have worse prognosis than tumors in the bladder lumen.
▶ T1 bladder cancer is limited to the subepithelial tissue, T2 is limited to the muscle layer, T3 represents extension into the perivesical fat, and T4 represents involvement of adjacent organs or pelvic sidewall.
▶ Lack of muscle wall results in higher incidence of stage 3 or higher tumors in diverticular tumors than in classic bladder TCC.
▶ On imaging, diverticular tumors appear as enhancing soft tissue nodules or filling defects within a bladder diverticulum.
▶ Stranding or mass-like extension into the adjacent fat suggests perivesical extension and is a poor prognostic sign.
▶ Approximately 33% of bladder diverticular TCCs are superficial at the time of diagnosis.

Management

▶ Cystoscopic excision is recommended for early disease. Chemotherapy, radiation, and surgery are recommended for more advanced disease. Surgical resection is the only curative approach if no distant metastatic disease is present.

Further Reading

Dondalski M, White EM, Ghahremani GG, Patel SK. Carcinoma arising in urinary bladder diverticula: imaging findings in six patients. *AJR Am J Roentgenol.* 1993;161(4):817–820.

History

▶ Incidental finding in a 57-year-old male

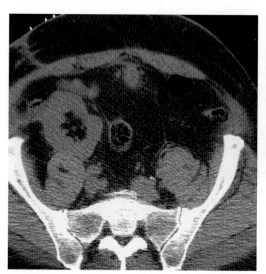

Figure 71.1

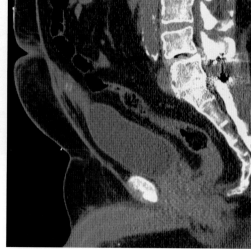

Figure 71.2

Case 71   Urachal Remnant

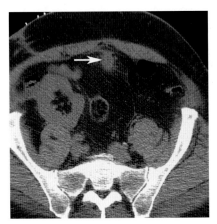

Figure 71.3

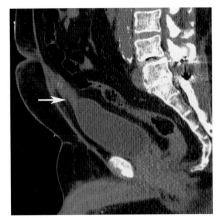

Figure 71.4

Findings

▶ Unenhanced axial and sagittal CT images (Figures 71.1 and 71.2) show a supravesical soft tissue attenuation lesion that extends from the anterior dome of the bladder to the umbilicus (arrow in Figures 71.3 and 71.4).

Differential Diagnosis

▶ The supravesical location of the lesion and extension from the bladder dome to the umbilicus are diagnostic of pathology involving the urachal remnant. Patent urachus (50%), urachal cyst (30%), umbilical-urachal sinus (15%), and vesico-urachal diverticulum (5%) are different types of congenital urachal anomalies. The solid mass–like configuration seen here is not compatible with an uncomplicated urachal cyst, diverticula, or sinus tract. The solid nature suggests either development of urachal malignancy or infection of a urachal remnant. Biopsy revealed inflammation in the urachal remnant without evidence of malignancy.

Teaching Points

▶ The urachus (or median umbilical ligament) is an embryological remnant of the genitourinary tract. It is a tubular structure that extends from the bladder dome to the umbilicus; it involutes before birth.

▶ A patent urachus has communication between the bladder and umbilicus and usually presents with urine discharge in neonates.

▶ A urachal cyst develops when the urachus closes at the bladder and the umbilicus but remains patent in between.

▶ Vesico-urachal diverticulum develops due to failure of closure of the urachus at the bladder end.

▶ Urachal remnants are susceptible to infection.

▶ The complex nature and heterogeneity of enhancement may make it difficult to differentiate an infected urachal remnant from urachal malignancy.

▶ Urachal adenocarcinoma represents 90% of urachal malignancies.

▶ Urachal adenocarcinoma represents 0.5% of all bladder cancers; however, 34% of bladder adenocarcinomas are of urachal origin.

Management

▶ Sampling to exclude malignancy; excision to prevent reinfection

Further Reading

Yu JS, Kim KW, Lee HJ, Lee YJ, Yoon CS, Kim MJ. Urachal remnant diseases: spectrum of CT and US findings. *Radiographics.* 2001;21(2):451–461.

History

▶ 53-year-old diabetic female with dysuria

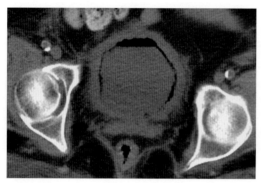

Figure 72.1

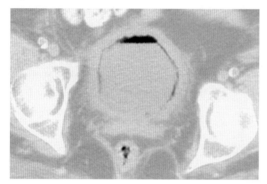

Figure 72.2

Case 72 Emphysematous Cystitis

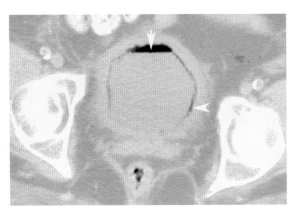

Figure 72.3

Findings

▶ Axial unenhanced CT images (Figures 72.1 and 72.2) through the bladder show multiple punctate foci of gas delineating the bladder wall (arrowhead in Figure 72.3). Intraluminal gas is also present (arrow).

Differential Diagnosis

▶ Differential diagnosis of gas within the bladder lumen includes recent instrumentation, fistula to the bowel, and infection. In this patient, the presence of gas in the bladder wall in addition to intraluminal gas is diagnostic of emphysematous cystitis.

Teaching Points

▶ Emphysematous cystitis is a complicated lower urinary tract infection that is characterized by gas within the wall and lumen of the bladder.
▶ It is the most common gas-forming infection of the urinary tract.
▶ Two thirds of patients with emphysematous cystitis are diabetics.
▶ Clinical presentation varies from asymptomatic to mild dysuria to severe sepsis.
▶ *Escherichia coli* and *Klebsiella pnemoniae* are the most common infecting organisms.
▶ Emphysematous cystitis has much better prognosis than emphysematous pyelonephritis.
▶ Mortality with emphysematous cystitis is approximately 7%.
▶ If not treated, infection may spread to the upper urinary tract, significantly increasing morbidity and mortality.

Management

▶ Patients are usually treated with intravenous antibiotics. Surgery may be needed in severe cases.

Further Reading

Thomas AA, Lane BR, Thomas AZ, Remer EM, Campbell SC, Shoskes DA. Emphysematous cystitis: a review of 135 cases. *BJU Int.* 2007;100(1):17–20.

Case 73

History

▸ Conventional cystogram (Figures 73.1 and 73.2) and CT cystogram (Figures 73.3 and 73.4) from two patients with hematuria following trauma

Figure 73.1

Figure 73.2

Figure 73.3

Figure 73.4

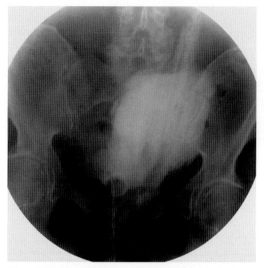

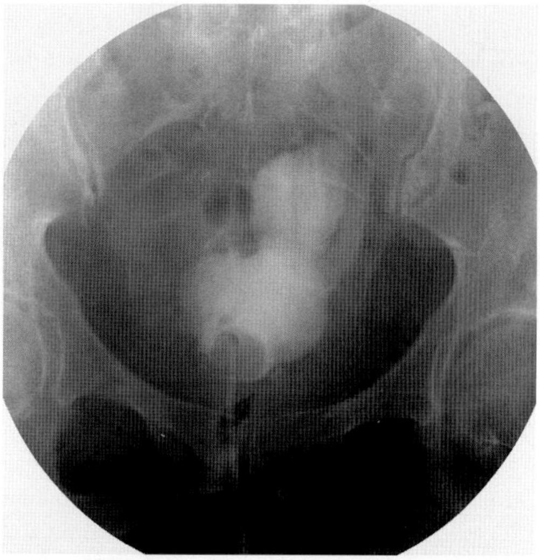

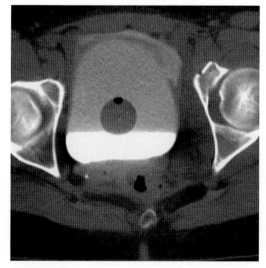

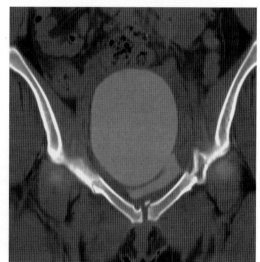

Case 73 Extraperitoneal Bladder Rupture

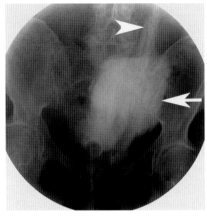

Figure 73.5

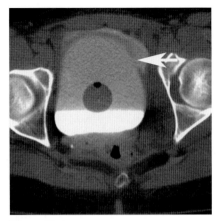

Figure 73.6

Findings

► Cystogram images (Figures 73.1 and 73.2) obtained after instillation of contrast through a Foley catheter show a partially distended bladder with streaky, flame-shaped extravasation of contrast into the perivesical space (arrow in Figure 73.5) and tracking along the abdominal wall (arrowhead in Figure 73.5).

► CT cystogram images (Figures 73.3 and 73.4) show contrast extravasation from the bladder into the anterior perivesical space through a rent in the inferior left anterolateral bladder wall (arrow in Figure 73.6). Pelvic fractures are identified.

Differential Diagnosis

► Identification of extravesical contrast during cystogram is consistent with bladder rupture. Bladder rupture can be extraperitoneal, intraperitoneal, or combined. On conventional cystogram, the streaky appearance of the extraluminal contrast is typical of extraperitoneal rupture. The extravasated contrast tracks cranially along the preperitoneal (extraperitoneal) space. This distribution is different from that of intraperitoneal rupture in which contrast outlines bowel loops and peritoneal spaces. The CT cystogram demonstrates extravasation into the anterior perivesical space, which is typical of extraperitoneal rupture and also identifies the site of rupture.

Teaching Points

► Extraperitoneal bladder rupture constitutes 80%–90% of bladder injury.
► About 80% of patients with bladder trauma have associated pelvic fractures.
► Up to 20% of patients with bladder injury have associated urethral injury.
► Bladder evaluation is indicated in patients with gross hematuria and pelvic fracture following trauma.
► CT cystography is performed after instillation of 350–400 cc of dilute contrast into the bladder.
► Extraperitoneal contrast tracks along fascial planes to the prevesical soft tissues, perineum, scrotum, thighs, and abdominal wall.
► Conventional and CT cystography both have 95% sensitivity and 100% specificity.
► Bladder neck injury is rare and requires early repair to prevent incontinence.

Management

► Most extraperitoneal bladder ruptures are managed conservatively with placement of catheter unless there is bladder neck injury.

Further Readings

Vaccaro JP, Brody JM. CT cystography in the evaluation of major bladder trauma. *Radiographics*. 2000;20(5):1373–1381.

ACR Appropriateness Criteria: suspected lower urinary tract trauma. http://www.acr.org/~/media/ACR/Documents/ AppCriteria/Diagnostic/SuspectedLowerUrinaryTractTrauma.pdf. Last accessed May 14, 2014

History

▶ 40-year-old male with hematuria after blunt trauma to abdomen

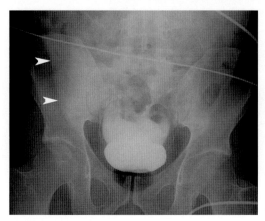

Figure 74.1

Case 74 Intraperitoneal Bladder Rupture

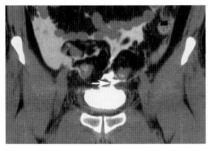
Figure 74.2

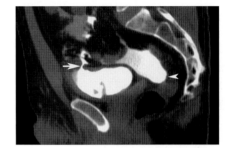
Figure 74.3

Findings

▶ Pelvic radiograph (Figure 74.1) obtained after administration of intravenous contrast demonstrates excreted contrast in the bladder. Radiopaque contrast superior to the bladder does not conform to the shape of the bladder and surrounds gas-filled bowel loops. Increased density delineates the right paracolic gutter (arrowheads).

▶ Coronal and sagittal CT cystogram images (Figures 74.2 and 74.3) obtained after instilling contrast through a Foley catheter show a rent in the bladder dome (arrow). The leaked contrast tracks around small bowel loops, delineating the paracolic gutters and rectovesical pouch (arrowhead).

Differential Diagnosis

▶ Presence of contrast outside a partially distended bladder on the pelvic radiograph is consistent with bladder injury. Distribution of the extravesical contrast determines extraperitoneal, intraperitoneal, or combined intraperitoneal–extraperitoneal nature of the injury. In this patient, extravesical contrast outlines intraperitoneal bowel and peritoneal recesses (paracolic gutter, rectovesical pouch), confirming an intraperitoneal bladder rupture. Absence of streaky contrast in the perivesical space or extension along fascial planes to the perineum, thigh, scrotum, or preperitoneal space excludes an extraperitoneal component of bladder injury. CT cystogram confirms the diagnosis by demonstrating a rent in the bladder dome, which is lined by peritoneum and is the usual site of intraperitoneal bladder injury.

Teaching Points

▶ Bladder injury is classified into type 1, simple bladder contusion (no radiologic abnormality); type 2, intraperitoneal rupture; type 3, interstitial bladder injury (contrast dissecting into bladder wall); type 4, extraperitoneal bladder rupture; and type 5, combined intra- and extraperitoneal bladder rupture.

▶ Intraperitoneal rupture constitutes 10%–20% of bladder injuries.

▶ Intraperitoneal bladder rupture occurs either due to a blow to a distended bladder that results in disruption of the superior peritoneal portion of the bladder wall or direct penetrating injury.

Management

▶ Intraperitoneal bladder rupture (unlike extraperitoneal injury) is always managed with surgical repair to prevent peritonitis.

Further Reading

1. Sandler CM, Hall JT, Rodriguez MB, Corriere JN Jr. Bladder injury in blunt pelvic trauma. *Radiology*. 1986;158(3):633–638.
2. ACR Appropriateness Criteria: suspected lower urinary tract trauma. http://www.acr.org/~/media/ACR/Documents/AppCriteria/Diagnostic/SuspectedLowerUrinaryTractTrauma.pdf. Last accessed May 14, 2014.

History

▶ 40-year-old female with fecal incontinence

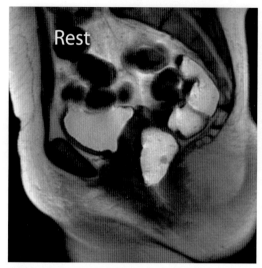

Figure 75.1

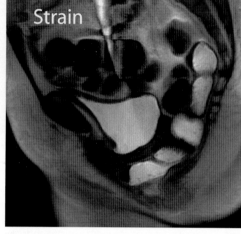

Figure 75.2

Case 75 Pelvic Organ Prolapse

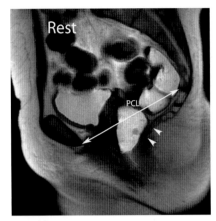

Figure 75.3

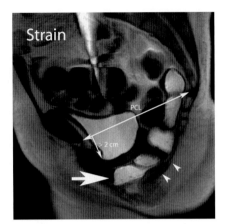

Figure 75.4

Findings

▶ Sagittal T2-weighted dynamic pelvic MR images were obtained during rest (Figure 75.1) and strain (Figure 75.2). Dynamic MR imaging uses measurements relative to the pubococcygeal line (PCL) drawn from the inferior edge of the pubis to the sacrococcygeal joint to assess pelvic organ prolapse.

▶ Bladder neck >2 cm below the PCL on the strain image (arrow in Figure 75.4) is consistent with a cystocele.

▶ Anterior protrusion of the anterior rectal wall (large arrow in Figure 75.4) is consistent with a rectocele.

▶ Levator plate (arrowheads in Figures 75.3 and 75.4) is the midline raphe of the iliococcygeus. Levator plate should be parallel to the PCL (as in Figure 75.3). Caudal angulation >10 to the PCL, as noted on the strain image (Figure 75.4), is consistent with weakness of the posterior compartment of the pelvic floor.

Differential Diagnosis

▶ Differential diagnosis of fecal incontinence includes neuromuscular disease, collagen vascular disease, or inflammatory bowel disease.

Teaching Points

▶ Weakness of the pelvic floor muscles, fascia, and ligaments cause abnormal descent of the bladder, uterovaginal vault, and rectum. This can result in urinary incontinence, fecal incontinence, and pelvic organ prolapse.

▶ Prolapse can affect the anterior compartment, which contains the bladder and urethra (cystocele); middle compartment, which contains the uterus and vagina (apical descent); or posterior compartment, which contains the rectum (rectocele or laxity).

▶ Multicompartment prolapse is common and commonly missed on physical exam.

▶ Pregnancy, multiparity, and advanced age are risk factors.

▶ Dynamic MR imaging is the most developed modality for assessing pelvic organ prolapse, but ultrasound is also being used.

▶ Evacuatory cine clips show more abnormalities than strain alone.

▶ Rectal gel helps distend the rectum, displaces gas and allows for evacuation phase.

▶ Levator tears can be unilateral or bilateral. Levator muscle injury correlates with fecal incontinence with or without prolapse.

Management

▶ If biofeedback is unsuccessful, transvaginal or open surgery is the treatment of choice.

Further Reading
Law YM, Fielding JR. MRI of pelvic floor dysfunction: review. *AJR Am J Roentgenol.* 2008;191(6 suppl):S45–53.

History

▶ Incidental finding in a 53-year-old male immigrant from Africa

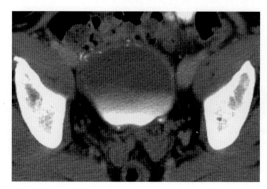

Figure 76.1

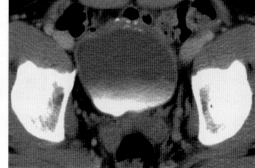

Figure 76.2

Case 76   Bladder Wall Calcification

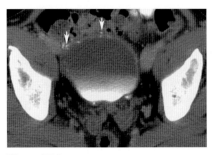 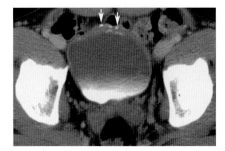

Figure 76.3   **Figure 76.4**

Findings

▶ Axial contrast-enhanced CT images through the pelvis (Figures 76.1 and 76.2) show bladder wall thickening with multiple foci of curvilinear and nodular bladder wall calcification (arrows in Figures 76.3 and 76.4).

Differential Diagnosis

▶ Differential diagnosis of bladder wall calcification includes urothelial carcinoma, schistosomiasis, tuberculosis, cyclophosphamide-induced cystitis, and radiation cystitis. In urothelial carcinoma, nodular calcification is associated with soft tissue masses and can be excluded here. Bladder tuberculosis is typically associated with thick-walled, small-capacity "thimble" bladder in a patient with sterile pyuria. Cyclophosphamide- and radiation-induced cystitis have typical antecedent history. Schitosomiasis is endemic in parts of Africa and causes bladder wall thickening with curvilinear calcifications. The diagnosis of schistosomiasis was confirmed in this patient by urine analysis.

Teaching Points

▶ Although uncommon in the United States, schistosomiasis is the most common cause of bladder wall calcification in the world.
▶ Genitourinary infection is caused by *Schistosoma haematobium*.
▶ Deposition of eggs in bladder wall veins incites chronic granulomatous inflammation. Chronic inflammation is a predisposing factor for squamous cell carcinoma.
▶ Bladder calcifications represent calcified schistosoma eggs.
▶ Tuberculous cystitis is due to spread of infection from the upper tracts. Concomitant upper tract changes are often present with bladder infection. Bladder involvement leads to fibrosis and reduction in bladder volume, in turn, causing urinary frequency.
▶ Radiation and chemotherapy cause hemorrhagic cystitis. Calcification is a rare finding.

Management

▶ Cystoscopy to exclude malignancy

Further Reading
Wong-You-Cheong JJ, Woodward PJ, Manning MA, Davis CJ. From the archives of the AFIP: inflammatory and nonneoplastic bladder masses: radiologic-pathologic correlation. *Radiographics*. 2006;26(6):1847–1868.

Section V   Prostate

History

► 65-year-old male with difficulty voiding

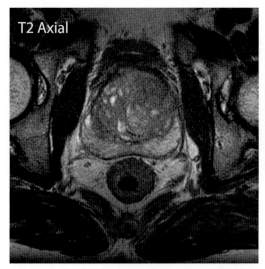

Figure 77.1

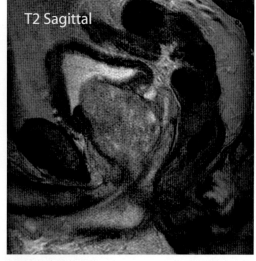

Figure 77.2

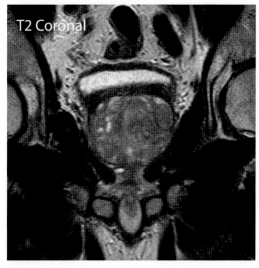

Figure 77.3

Case 77 Benign Prostatic Hyperplasia

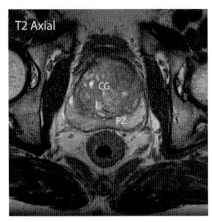

Figure 77.4

Findings

▶ Axial, sagittal, and coronal T2-weighted images of the prostate gland (Figures 77.1–77.3) demonstrate an enlarged heterogeneous predominantly T2 hypointense central gland (CG in Figure 77.4) with small T2 hyperintense areas. The peripheral zone (PZ in Figure 77.4) is homogeneously T2 hyperintense without any focal lesion. Protrusion of the enlarged prostate into the bladder base is noted on the sagittal image.

Differential Diagnosis

▶ Heterogeneous enlargement of the central gland seen here is characteristic of benign prostatic hyperplasia (BPH). Prostate cancer commonly affects the peripheral zone and is identified as T2 hypointense areas within the T2 hyperintense peripheral zone of the gland.

Teaching Points

▶ BPH starts in the transitional zone that surrounds the urethra.
▶ Clinical symptoms of BPH are caused by compression of the bladder neck and urethra by the enlarged gland.
▶ Enlargement of the subvesicular part of the prostate may cause protrusion into the bladder base.
▶ On MRI, the benign hypertrophied part of the gland is often separated from the peripheral zone by a pseudocapsule.
▶ BPH is usually diagnosed by clinical evaluation; MRI is not a part of the diagnostic work-up.
▶ In patients with BPH, ultrasound is used to evaluate the kidneys, assess post-void residual in the bladder, and obtain volume of the prostate gland.

Management

▶ Transurethral or open resection

Further Reading

Grossfeld GD, Coakley FV. Benign prostatic hyperplasia: clinical overview and value of diagnostic imaging. *Radiol Clin North Am.* 2000;38(1):31–47.

History

▶ 66-year-old male with biopsy-proven prostate cancer

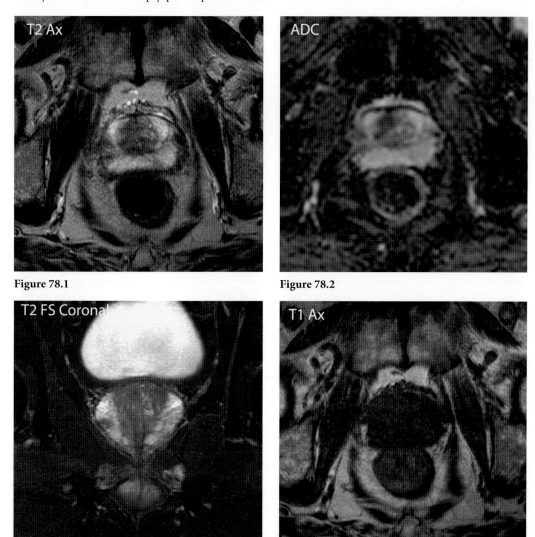

Figure 78.1

Figure 78.2

Figure 78.3

Figure 78.4

Case 78   Prostate Cancer with Extracapsular Spread

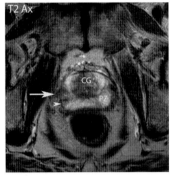

Figure 78.5

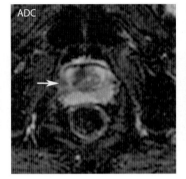

Figure 78.6

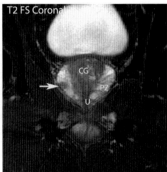

Figure 78.7

Findings

▶ Axial T2-weighted image through the mid prostate gland (Figures 78.1 and 78.5) shows a T2 hypointense focus in the right lateral aspect peripheral zone (arrow in Figure 78.5, CG, central gland; PZ, peripheral zone) that is causing an irregular bulge in the prostatic contour. The thin T2 hypointense line representing the normal prostatic capsule (arrowhead in Figure 78.5) is obliterated at this location.

▶ The lesion is hypointense on the corresponding apparent diffusion coefficient map (Figure 78.2, arrow in Figure 78.6), suggesting restricted diffusion.

▶ Fat-suppressed T2-weighted coronal image (Figures 78.3 and 78.7) depicts the T2 hypointense area in the right lateral peripheral mid gland (arrow in Figure 78.7; U, urethra).

▶ T1-weighted image (Figure 78.4) does not show any signal abnormality within the gland.

Differential Diagnosis

▶ T2 hypointense focus in the peripheral zone of the prostate with corresponding diffusion restriction is consistent with prostate cancer. The bulge in the prostatic contour with focal obliteration of the capsule indicates extracapsular extension. Stage T1 and T2 prostate cancer is confined to the gland. Extracapsular extension (as seen here) and seminal vesicle involvement represent T3 disease. Invasion of other adjacent organs is T4 disease.

Teaching Points

▶ Normal prostate consists of a homogeneously T2 hyperintense peripheral zone and a heterogeneous signal central gland.

▶ Seventy percent of prostate cancer arises in the peripheral zone.

▶ Prostate cancer is identified as T2 hypointense foci within the hyperintense peripheral zone.

▶ Focal irregular prostate contour bulge, asymmetry/encasement of neurovascular bundle (at 5 and 7 o' clock positions), obliteration of rectoprostatic angle, and low T2 signal in the seminal vesicle suggest extraglandular tumor invasion.

▶ Restricted diffusion, increased choline-to-citrate ratio on spectroscopy, and early hyperenhancement with rapid washout on dynamic contrast-enhanced MRI are all indicative of prostate cancer.

Management

▶ Prostatectomy for disease limited to prostate; hormone ablation/radiotherapy for extraglandular extension

Further Reading

Verma S, Rajesh A. A clinically relevant approach to imaging prostate cancer: review. *AJR Am J Roentgenol.* 2011;196(3 suppl):S1–10.

History

▶ 70-year-old male with biopsy-proven prostate cancer

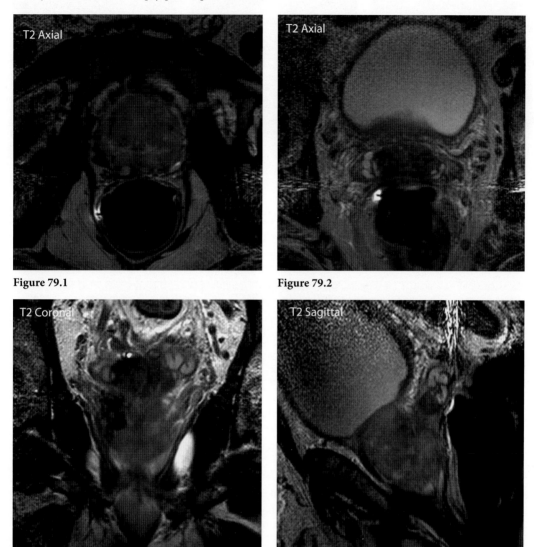

Figure 79.1

Figure 79.2

Figure 79.3

Figure 79.4

Case 79 Prostate Cancer with Seminal Vesicle and Neurovascular Bundle Involvement

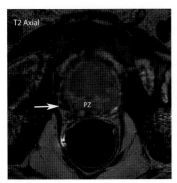

Figure 79.5

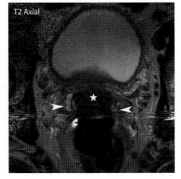

Figure 79.6

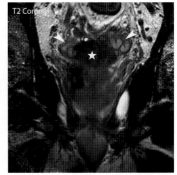

Figure 79.7

Findings

▸ Axial T2-weighted image through the prostate base (Figure 79.1) shows diffuse abnormal heterogeneous decreased signal intensity throughout the peripheral zone with multiple areas of contour bulges in the prostatic outline (black arrowhead in Figure 79.5). Enlargement of the right neurovascular bundle is noted (arrow in Figure 79.5).

▸ Axial, coronal, and sagittal T2-weighted images through the seminal vesicles (Figures 79.2–79.4) show contiguous areas of decreased T2 signal intensity extending from the prostate base to the bilateral seminal vesicles (asterisk). The seminal vesicles maintain their normal architecture and high T2 signal peripherally (white arrowheads in Figures 79.6 and 79.7).

Differential Diagnosis

▸ Areas of decreased T2 signal in the peripheral zone are consistent with prostate malignancy. The disease is particularly extensive and diffuse in this patient. Multiple areas of contour bulges are concerning for extracapsular spread. The enlargement of the right neurovascular bundle at the 7 o'clock position suggests involvement by the malignancy. The T2 low signal infiltrating into the medial aspect of the seminal vesicles, which are normally T2 hyperintense tubular structures, is consistent with seminal vesicle involvement.

Teaching Points

▸ Prostate MRI is the most accurate noninvasive method of locally staging prostate cancer.

▸ Prostate cancer appears as areas of low T2 signal in contrast to the normally T2 hyperintense peripheral zone.

▸ Hemorrhage, prostatitis, and post-hormone/radiation therapy changes are nonmalignant causes of low T2 signal in the peripheral zone. Correlation with T1-weighted imaging and techniques such as diffusion-weighted imaging, spectroscopy, and dynamic contrast enhancement help increase specificity.

Management

▸ Prostatectomy for disease limited to the gland, and hormone ablation/radiation for disease extending beyond the gland

Further Reading

Bonekamp D, Jacobs MA, El-Khouli R, Stoianovici D, Macura KJ. Advancements in MR imaging of the prostate: from diagnosis to interventions. *Radiographics*. 2011;31(3):677–703.

History

▶ 58-year-old diabetic male with dysuria and perineal pain; images from pelvic CT on presentation (Figure 80.1) and follow-up MR after 7 days (Figures 80.2–80.4)

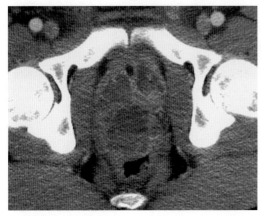

Figure 80.1

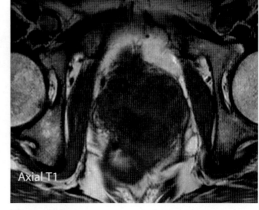

Figure 80.2

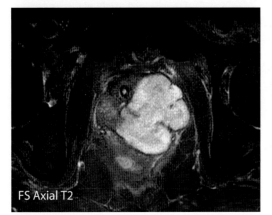

Figure 80.3

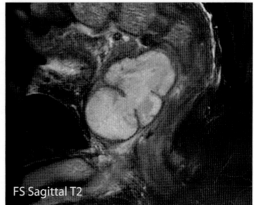

Figure 80.4

Case 80 Prostate Abscess

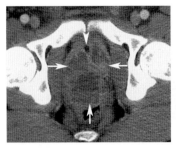

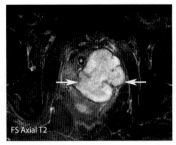

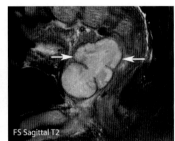

Figure 80.5   **Figure 80.6**   **Figure 80.7**

Findings

▶ Contrast-enhanced CT (Figure 80.1) shows a large rim-enhancing low-attenuation lesion involving the prostate (arrows in Figure 80.5). A Foley catheter is present in the prostatic urethra (arrowhead).

▶ Axial T1-weighted (Figure 80.2) and T2-weighted (Figure 80.3) MRI images at the level of the mid prostate gland show a T1 hypointense and T2 hyperintense lobulated cystic lesion (arrows in Figure 80.6) with internal septations that involve the central and peripheral zones of the prostate and extend into the periprostatic tissues.

▶ Sagittal T2-weighted image through the prostate (Figure 80.4) shows the craniocaudal extent of the T2 hyperintense cystic lesion (arrows in Figure 80.7).

Differential Diagnosis

▶ Differential diagnosis of cystic lesions of the prostate includes congenital utricle and mullerian duct cysts, ejaculatory duct cyst, cystic degeneration of benign prostatic hypertrophy, and prostatic abscess. Prostatic utricle and mullerian duct cysts are both midline cysts. Ejaculatory duct cysts are along the course of the ejaculatory duct just lateral to the midline in the central zone. Cystic degeneration of benign prostatic hyperplasia is limited to the central gland. Prostate abscesses occur anywhere in the gland and may have extraglandular spread. Presence of a large cystic prostatic lesion with thick enhancing walls and internal septations is consistent with a prostate abscess in this patient with clinical symptoms of infection.

Teaching Points

▶ Prostatic abscesses can present with fever, dysuria, urinary frequency, and perineal pain. A soft fluctuant prostate may be palpated on digital examination.

▶ Predisposing factors include diabetes, immunosuppression, and permanent catheterization.

▶ On ultrasound, prostatic abscesses appear as hypoechoic collections with debris, septations, and increased perilesional vascularity.

▶ CT and MRI demonstrate extraglandular extension often underestimated on ultrasound.

▶ Prostatic abscesses can form fistulas to the bladder, urethra, rectum, or perineum.

Management

▶ Ultrasound-guided drainage and antibiotics

Further Reading

Barozzi L, Pavlica P, Menchi I, De Matteis M, Canepari M. Prostatic abscess: diagnosis and treatment. *AJR Am J Roentgenol.* 1998;170(3):753–757.

History

▶ 50-year-old male with renal failure and pelvic pain

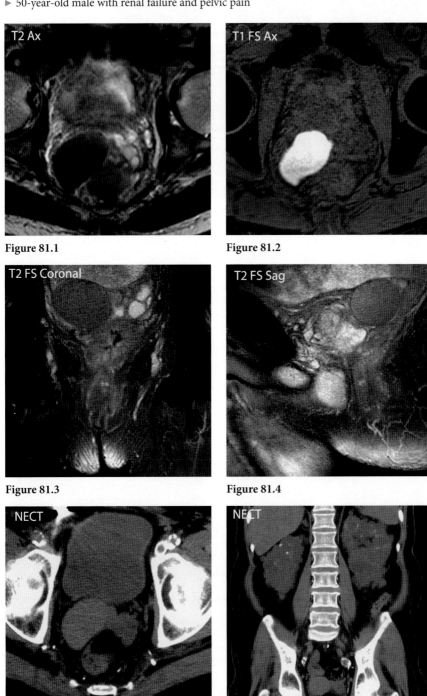

Figure 81.1

Figure 81.2

Figure 81.3

Figure 81.4

Figure 81.5

Figure 81.6

Case 81 Seminal Vesicle Cyst

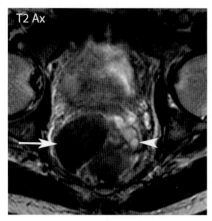
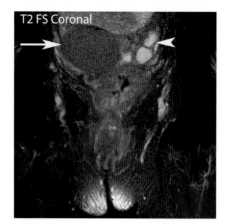

Figure 81.7   **Figure 81.8**

Findings

▶ Axial T2-weighted (Figure 81.1), axial fat-suppressed T1-weighted (Figure 81.2), and fat-suppressed T2-weighted coronal (Figure 81.3) and sagittal (Figure 81.4) images show a well-defined lesion in the expected region of the right seminal vesicle. The lesion is hypointense on T2-weighted imaging (arrow in Figures 81.7 and 81.8) and very homogeneously hyperintense on T1-weighted imaging. The left seminal vesicle is mildly dilated but otherwise unremarkable (arrowhead in Figures 81.7 and 81.8).

▶ Unenhanced axial and coronal CT images (Figures 81.5 and 81.6) show the lesion to be hyperdense compared to the left seminal vesicle. Coronal image shows innumerable bilateral renal cysts.

Differential Diagnosis

▶ Homogeneous high signal intensity on T1-weighted fat-suppressed imaging and low signal intensity on T2-weighted imaging are consistent with a hemorrhagic cyst. The cyst replaces the right seminal vesicle, helping to differentiate it from prostatic or vas deferens cysts, which can occur in this vicinity. Innumerable bilateral renal cysts are consistent with autosomal dominant polycystic kidney disease. Polycystic kidney disease is often associated with seminal vesicle cysts, and its presence helps confirm the diagnosis.

Teaching Points

▶ Seminal vesicle cysts occur in 40%–60% patients with autosomal dominant polycystic kidney disease.
▶ Congenital seminal vesicle cysts are associated with other genitourinary anomalies, most commonly ipsilateral renal aplasia.
▶ Seminal vesicle cysts are often asymptomatic but may present with hematuria, dysuria, or hematospermia.
▶ Hemorrhage into seminal vesicle cyst is associated with hematospermia.

Management

▶ Excise only if symptomatic

Further Reading

Kim B, Kawashima A, Ryu JA, Takahashi N, Hartman RP, King BF Jr. Imaging of the seminal vesicle and vas deferens. *Radiographics.* 2009;29(4):1105–1121.

Section VI   Urethra, Vagina, and Penis

History

▶ 24-year-old male with hematuria following bicycle accident

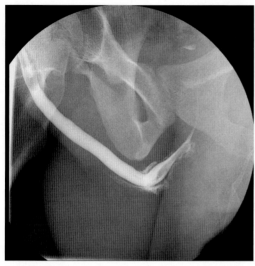

Figure 82.1

Case 82   Anterior Urethral Injury: Type V

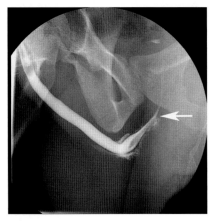

Figure 82.2

Findings

▶ Retrograde urethrogram (Figure 82.1) shows extravasation of contrast from the proximal bulbar urethra below the urogenital diaphragm (arrow in Figure 82.2) that tracks around the anterior urethra. Contrast is identified in the bladder. The bulbomembranous junction is identified by the cone of the bulbar urethra. In patients without good urethral distention it is identified by a virtual line connecting the inferior margins of the obturator foramina.

Differential Diagnosis

▶ A urethral tear can be isolated to the anterior urethra distal to the bulbomembranous junction (type V injury), involve prostatomembranous urethra with or without disruption of urogenital diaphragm (type II/III injury), or involve the bladder neck (type IV). In this patient, the site of contrast extravasation is in the bulbar urethra and the contrast tracks around the anterior urethra below the urogenital diaphragm, confirming an isolated anterior urethral or type V injury. Type II posterior urethral injury has extravasation limited to above the urogenital diaphragm, while type III injury has extravasation both above and below the urogenital diaphragm. Passage of contrast into the bladder suggests a partial tear in this patient.

Teaching Points

▶ Most anterior urethral injuries following blunt trauma involve the bulbar urethra.
▶ Straddle type injuries (bicycle accidents, falling on a pole) crush the bulbar urethra against the inferior pubic rami.
▶ Unlike posterior urethral injury, anterior urethral straddle injury is not usually associated with pelvic fractures and may initially have only mild symptoms.
▶ Delayed presentation due to bulbar stricture is common with straddle injury.
▶ Penetrating trauma, iatrogenic injury during catheterization, and penile fracture are other causes of anterior urethral injury.
▶ On urethrogram, the extravasated contrast is usually limited to the penile shaft by the Buck's fascia. Disruption of Buck's fascia due to severe straddle injury can cause contrast extravasation into the perineum deep to the Colles' fascia.

Management

▶ Conservative

Further Reading
Rosenstein DI, Alsikafi NF. Diagnosis and classification of urethral injuries. *Urol Clin North Am.* 2006;33(1):73–85, vi–vii.

History

▶ 28-year-old male with blood at urethral meatus following motor vehicle accident

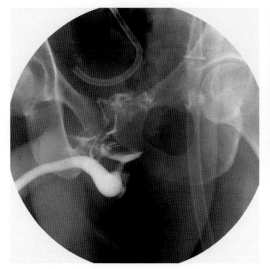

Figure 83.1

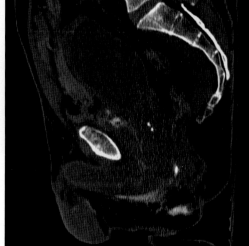

Figure 83.2

Case 83 Urethral Injury: Type III

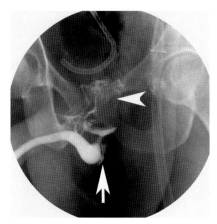

Figure 83.3

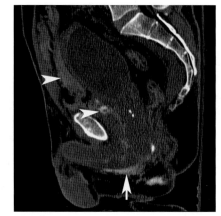

Figure 83.4

Findings

▶ Retrograde urethrogram (Figures 83.1 and 83.3) shows contrast extravasation from the urethra above the urogenital diaphragm (arrowhead) and below the urogenital diaphragm along the bulbar urethra (arrow). No contrast is seen in the bladder.

▶ Sagittal CT reconstruction imaging performed after retrograde urethrogram (Figures 83.2 and 83.4) shows residual contrast from the urethrogram above the urogenital diaphragm posterior to the pubic symphysis and in the anterior prevesical space (arrowheads) as well as below the urogenital diaphragm around the penile shaft (arrow).

Differential Diagnosis

▶ Contrast extravasation above and below the urogenital diaphragm noted on retrograde urethrogram is consistent with a type III posterior urethral injury. In type III injury, a membranous urethral tear is associated with urogenital diaphragm disruption and extends into the proximal bulbar urethra. Lack of any contrast in the bladder is concerning for a complete tear in this patient. Type II urethral injury involves the membranous urethra but spares the urogenital diaphragm and results in contrast extravasation above the urogenital diaphragm. Type IV injury involves the bladder neck. In this patient, the bladder neck is not opacified and cannot be assessed. Cystography is required to evaluate for associated bladder injury.

Teaching Points

▶ Type II and type III urethral injuries are usually associated with pelvic fractures.
▶ Type III urethral injury constitutes 66%–85% of all posterior urethral injuries.
▶ Type I and type II injuries each constitute 10%–15% of posterior urethral injuries.
▶ Complete tear is more common than partial tear in type II and type III injuries.
▶ Partial posterior urethral tears often heal without stricture formation; however, complete tears almost always heal with stricturing.

Management

▶ Urinary diversion with suprapubic catheter; resulting stricture is treated with urethroplasty electively

Further Reading

Rosenstein DI, Alsikafi NF. Diagnosis and classification of urethral injuries. *Urol Clin North Am*. 2006;33(1):73–85, vi–vii.
ACR Appropriateness Criteria: suspected lower urinary tract trauma. http://www.acr.org/~/media/ACR/Documents/ AppCriteria/Diagnostic/SuspectedLowerUrinaryTractTrauma.pdf

History

▶ 37-year-old male with hematuria after motor vehicle accident

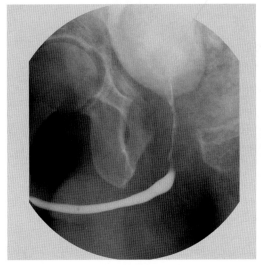

Figure 84.1

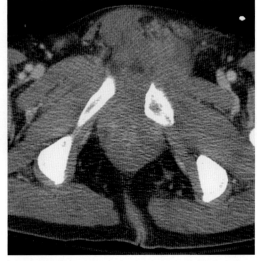

Figure 84.2

Case 84   Urethral Injury: Type I

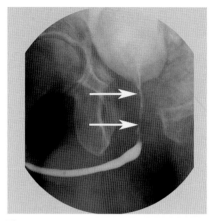

Figure 84.3

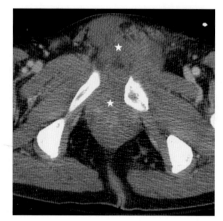

Figure 84.4

Findings

▶ Retrograde urethrogram (Figure 84.1) demonstrates a stretched but intact posterior urethra (arrows in Figure 84.3). No extravasation of contrast is seen. Pubic diastasis is present.

▶ Axial CT image (Figure 84.2) at the level of the prostate apex shows a large periprostatic hematoma that extends into subcutaneous tissues (asterisks in Figure 84.4) and obliterates periprostatic fat planes.

Differential Diagnosis

▶ Stretching of posterior urethra on retrograde urethrogram without contrast extravasation is characteristic of type I urethral injury in a patient with pelvic trauma. In type I injury, rupture of puboprostatic ligaments with periprostatic hematoma formation (seen in Figure 84.2) can result in significant stretching without tear of membranous urethra. Type II urethral injury is due to posterior urethral rupture above an intact urogenital diaphragm and causes contrast extravasation above the urogenital diaphragm. Type III urethral injury is due to injury of the prostatomembranous urethra with disruption of the urogenital diaphragm extending to the proximal anterior urethra and causes contrast extravasation both above and below the urogenital diaphragm. Type IV refers to bladder neck injury and type V refers to isolated anterior urethral injury.

Teaching Points

▶ Retrograde urethrography is the best initial study for suspected urethral injury and should be performed before catheterization in patients with blood at the meatus.

▶ Posterior urethral injuries are present in 4%–14% patients with pelvic fractures.

▶ Male posterior urethral injuries are due to shearing forces at the prostatomembranous junction that result in avulsion of the prostatic apex from the urogenital diaphragm.

▶ Urethral injury is uncommon in women due to its short length and relative mobility.

Management

▶ Suprapubic catheter placement and supportive care

Further Reading

Kawashima A, Sandler CM, Wasserman NF, LeRoy AJ, King BF Jr, Goldman SM. Imaging of urethral disease: a pictorial review. *Radiographics*. 2004;24(suppl) 1:S195–216.

History

▶ 35-year-old man with decreased urine flow

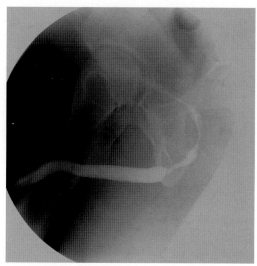

Figure 85.1

Urethra Injuries
─────────────────────

I: membranous urethra is
Stretched, periurethral hematoma
rupture of Pubo-prostatic ligaments
No contrast extravasation

II: Rupture above the UGD, intact UGD
Extraperitoneal Contrast
Post urethra Injury

III Rupture of prostatomemb urethra
with UGD damage
Contrast above and below UGD

IV: Bladder neck injury extending
to urethra

V Isolated
Anterior urethra Injury

Case 85 Anterior Urethral Stricture

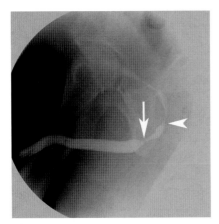

Figure 85.2

Findings

► Retrograde urethrogram (Figure 85.1) demonstrates a short-segment stricture in the bulbar part of the anterior urethra (arrow in Figure 85.2). Arrowhead in Figure 85.2 points to the conical tip of the bulbar urethra, which marks the bulbomembranous junction (urogenital diaphragm).

Differential Diagnosis

► Focal narrowing of the anterior urethra is consistent with a urethral stricture. Anterior urethral strictures can be traumatic, iatrogenic, or infectious in etiology. Straddle injury crushes the bulbar urethra and causes delayed development of bulbar urethral stricture. Iatrogenic strictures by indwelling catheters/instrumentation occur due to pressure necrosis, typically at the bulbomembranous region and penoscrotal junction. Gonococcal urethritis typically causes long-segment irregular anterior urethral strictures. In this patient, the bulbar urethral stricture was secondary to remote straddle injury.

Teaching Points

► The male urethra is 17.5–20 cm long and divided into anterior and posterior segments.
► The anterior urethra extends from just below the urogenital diaphragm to the urethral meatus. It is divided into bulbar and penile parts at the penoscrotal junction. The bulbar urethra extends from the urogenital diaphragm to the penoscrotal junction, and the penile urethra extends from the penoscrotal junction to the meatus.
► The posterior urethra is divided into prostatic and membranous segments. The prostatic urethra extends from the internal bladder sphincter to the verumonatum. The membranous urethra (1–1.5 cm) extends from the verumonatum to the external sphincter at the urogenital diaphragm.
► Urethral strictures commonly occur in males. Straddle injury is the most common external traumatic cause of anterior urethral stricture.
► Anterior urethral strictures are more common than posterior urethral strictures.
► Posterior urethral strictures are secondary to pelvic fractures or prostatic surgery.
► Retrograde urethrography is the primary imaging modality for evaluation of urethral strictures.
► Urethral strictures can result in the formation of periurethral abscesses that may drain externally and form urethroperineal fistulas.

Management

► Surgery for clinically significant stricture

Further Reading

Kawashima A, Sandler CM, Wasserman NF, LeRoy AJ, King BF Jr, Goldman SM. Imaging of urethral disease: a pictorial review. *Radiographics*. 2004;24(suppl) 1:S195–216.

History

▶ 65-year old male with history of radiation for prostate cancer (Figure 86.1) and 35-year-old male with history of gunshot wound to pelvis (Figure 86.2)

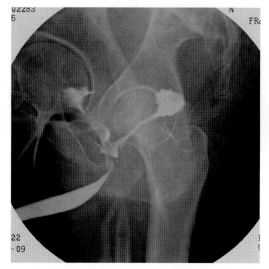

Figure 86.1

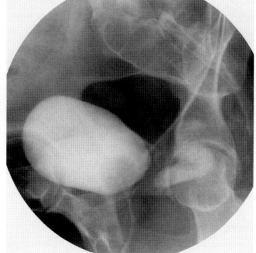

Figure 86.2

Case 86　Urinary Tract Fistula

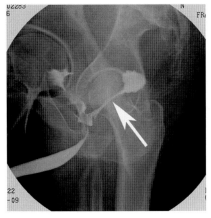

Figure 86.3

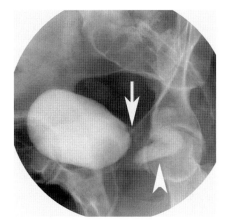

Figure 86.4

Findings

▶ Retrograde urethrogram image (Figure 86.1) shows opacification of the urethra, with contrast reaching the bladder. A linear contrast-filled track (arrow in Figure 86.3) extends posteriorly from the posterior urethra and partially fills the rectum.

▶ Figure 86.2 is a cystogram image from a different patient. The bladder is distended with contrast. A contrast-filled track (arrow in Figure 86.4) extends from the posterior bladder to the rectum and opacifies it (arrowhead).

Differential Diagnosis

▶ On retrograde urethrogram, the linear contrast-filled tract extending posteriorly from the posterior urethra to the rectum is consistent with a rectourethral fistula. The cystogram for the second patient shows a contrast-filled track from the bladder to the rectum that is consistent with a vesicorectal fistula.

Teaching Points

▶ Rectourethral fistula can be congenital or acquired. Congenital rectourethral fistulas present in neonates and are associated with imperforate anus.

▶ In adults, rectourethral fistulas are secondary to prostate surgery, radiation for prostate cancer, or instrumentation.

▶ Fistulas from bladder to bowel are commonly due to diverticular disease, tumors, inflammatory bowel disease, trauma, surgery, and radiation.

▶ Colovesical fistulas are commonly due to diverticular disease; ileovesical fistulas are usually due to Crohn's disease; and rectovesical fistulas are often due to trauma or neoplasm.

▶ Bladder fistulas are evaluated by CT, which demonstrates bladder air, or cystography. Delayed CT may show fistula tract.

▶ Urethral fistula are evaluated by retrograde urethrogram or voiding cystourethrogram.

Management

▶ Conservative management with percutaneous urinary diversion may heal small fistulas. Surgery is required for refractory cases.

Further Reading
Yu NC, Raman SS, Patel M, Barbaric Z. Fistulas of the genitourinary tract: a radiologic review. *Radiographics*. 2004;24(5):1331–1352.

Case 87

History

- 43-year-old woman with dysuria and post-void dribbling

)5464
)
M1
FRAME
30
-11
L =
W =
SP

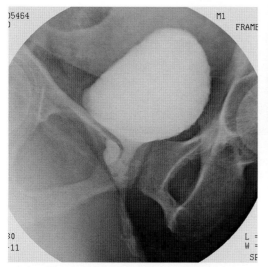

Figure 87.1

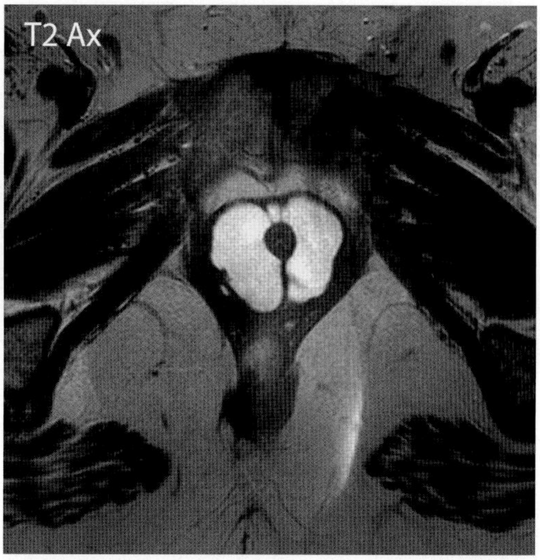

T2 Ax

Figure 87.2

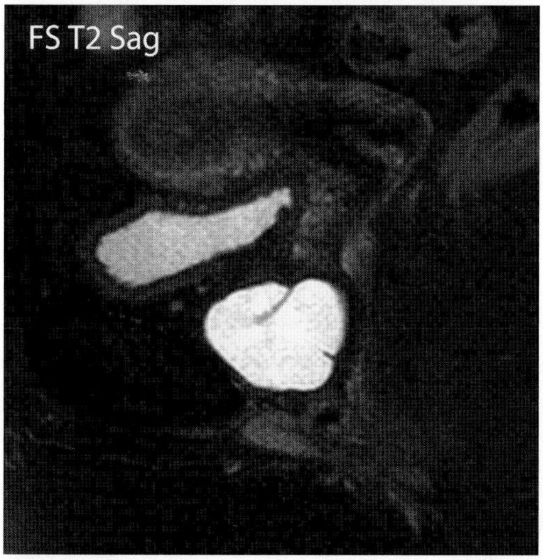

FS T2 Sag

Figure 87.3

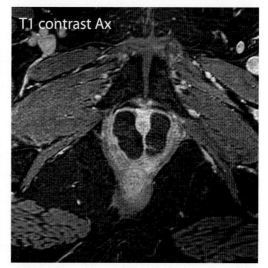

T1 contrast Ax

Figure 87.4

Case 87 Urethral Diverticulum

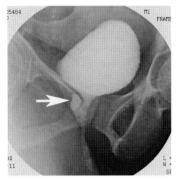
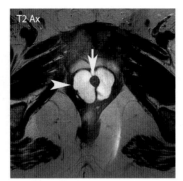

Figure 87.5   **Figure 87.6**

Findings

▶ Voiding cystourethrogram (Figures 87.1 and 87.5) shows contrast-filled outpouching communicating with the posterolateral urethra (arrow).

▶ Axial T2-weighted MR image (Figures 87.2 and 87.6) shows a T2 hyperintense cystic structure (arrowhead) encircling the urethra (arrow).

▶ Sagittal T2-weighted fat-suppressed image (Figure 87.3) shows the cystic structure to be anterior to the vagina in the region of mid urethra. Thin septations are present.

▶ Axial contrast-enhanced T1-weighted image (Figure 87.4) shows symmetric mild wall enhancement without any nodularity.

Differential Diagnosis

▶ Differential diagnosis here includes urethral diverticulum and other periurethral cystic lesions such as Gartner duct cyst, Bartholin gland cyst, Skene duct cyst, and Nabothian cyst. Gartner duct cyst can be excluded as it involves the anterolateral wall of the vagina and the vaginal wall is not involved in this patient. Bartholin gland cyst involves the posterior labia majora and can be excluded here. Skene duct cyst, although periurethral, is located lateral to external urethral meatus and not in the mid urethral region. Nabothian cyst involves the cervical stroma. The location of this cystic structure at the level of mid urethra, close relation to the urethra, and communication with the urethra are diagnostic of urethral diverticulum.

Teaching Points

▶ Urethral diverticula are focal outpouchings from the urethra seen predominantly in women.

▶ Incidence is mainly in the third through fifth decades.

▶ Diverticula develop due to obstruction and rupture of periurethral glands into the urethral lumen.

▶ Clinical presentation includes recurrent urinary tract infections, dysuria, and post-void dribbling.

▶ Typical location is in the posterolateral aspect of the mid urethra.

▶ Voiding cystourethrogram has 85% accuracy but is cumbersome. It may not opacify diverticula if the neck is not patent.

▶ MRI not only evaluates diverticula and contents but also identifies other diagnoses that may clinically mimic diverticula.

▶ Urinary stasis within diverticula can cause infection, stone formation, or malignancy.

Management

▶ Transvaginal diverticulectomy

Further Reading
Chaudhari VV, Patel MK, Douek M, Raman SS. MR imaging and US of female urethral and periurethral disease. *Radiographics*. 2010;30(7):1857–1874.

History

▶ 35-year-old woman with dysuria

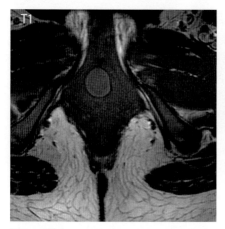

Figure 88.1

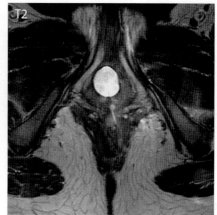

Figure 88.2

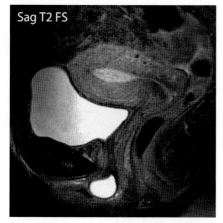

Figure 88.3

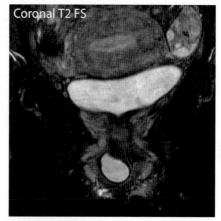

Figure 88.4

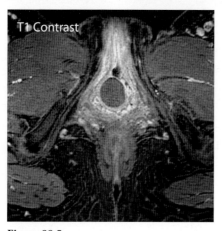

Figure 88.5

Case 88 Skene Duct Cyst

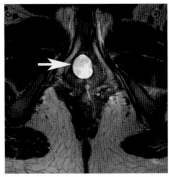
Figure 88.6

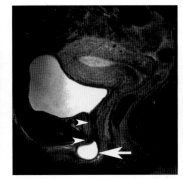
Figure 88.7

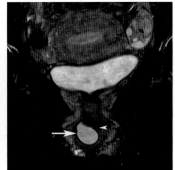
Figure 88.8

Findings

▶ Axial T1-weighted (Figure 88.1) and T2-weighted (Figure 88.2) images show a well-defined T1 hypointense and T2 hyperintense cyst near the external urethral meatus. Sagittal (Figure 88.3) and coronal (Figure 88.4) T2-weighted fat-suppressed images show that the distal most urethra is displaced laterally and anteriorly (arrowheads in Figures 88.7 and 88.8) by the cyst (arrow in Figures 88.6–88.8). No obvious communication with urethra is identified. Fat-suppressed contrast-enhanced axial T1-weighted image (Figure 88.5) does not show any nodularity or enhancement within the cyst.

Differential Diagnosis

▶ Differential diagnosis of a periurethral cystic lesion includes urethral diverticulum, Skene duct cyst, Gartner duct cyst, and Bartholin gland cyst. Gartner duct cyst can be excluded as it involves the anterolateral wall of the vagina and the vaginal wall is not involved in this patient. Bartholin gland cyst involves the posterior labia majora and can also be excluded. Skene duct cyst and urethral diverticulum both have the periurethral location noted in this patient. Urethral diverticula are typically located adjacent to the mid urethra and communicate with the urethra. Location adjacent to the external urethral meatus is typical of a Skene duct cyst, which is the favored diagnosis here.

Teaching Points

▶ Ducts of Skene secrete mucus into the distal urethra adjacent to the external urethral meatus.
▶ Periurethral cystic lesions, including Skene duct cysts, need to be differentiated from urethral diverticula.
▶ Urethral diverticula communicate with the urethra, while other periurethral cysts do not.

Management

▶ Excision if symptomatic

Further Reading
Chaudhari VV, Patel MK, Douek M, Raman SS. MR imaging and US of female urethral and periurethral disease. *Radiographics*. 2010;30(7):1857–1874.

History

▶ 47-year-old male with firm penile nodule

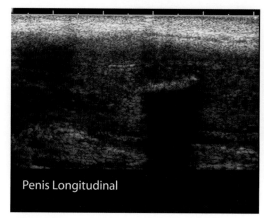

Penis Longitudinal

Figure 89.1

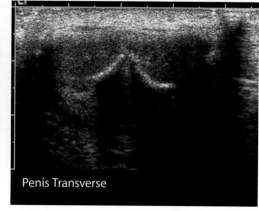

Penis Transverse

Figure 89.2

Case 89 Peyronie's Disease

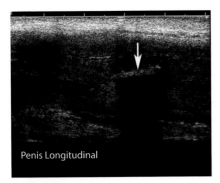

Penis Longitudinal

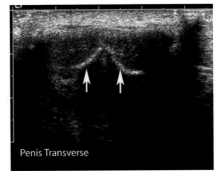

Penis Transverse

Figure 89.3

Figure 89.4

Findings

▸ Longitudinal and transverse ultrasound images (Figures 89.1 and 89.2) show linear shadowing calcified plaques involving the tunica albuginea (arrows in Figures 89.3 and 89.4).

Differential Diagnosis

▸ The linear calcifications along the tunica albuginea noted here are suggestive of calcified plaques seen in Peyronie's disease. Penile tumors present as irregular soft tissue masses on ultrasound. A penile foreign body can appear as a linear shadowing structure on ultrasound, but suggestive history is usually available.

Teaching Points

▸ Peyronie's disease is characterized by formation of fibrous tissue plaques within the tunica albuginea. Plaque formation causes penile deformity.
▸ Etiology is unclear but may be due to microtrauma and subsequent aberrant scar formation.
▸ Penile deformity, palpable plaques, and pain are presenting complaints.
▸ Peyronie's disease has an acute inflammatory stage followed by stabilization of symptoms.
▸ Ultrasound is used to identify the extent and location of palpable and nonpalpable plaques.
▸ Plaques are identified as areas of focal hyperechoic thickening of the tunica albuginea with associated shadowing. Plaque calcifications are associated with disease stabilization.
▸ On MRI, plaques appear as T1 and T2 hypointense areas in the tunica.

Management

▸ Conservative treatment in acute phase; surgery after disease stabilization for severe penile deformity

Further Reading
Kalokairinou K, Konstantinidis C, Domazou M, Kalogeropoulos T, Kosmidis P, Gekas A. US imaging in Peyronie's disease. *J Clin Imaging Sci.* 2012;2:63.

History

▶ 70-year-old man for staging of penile cancer

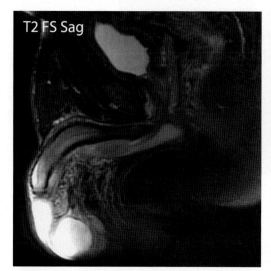

Figure 90.1

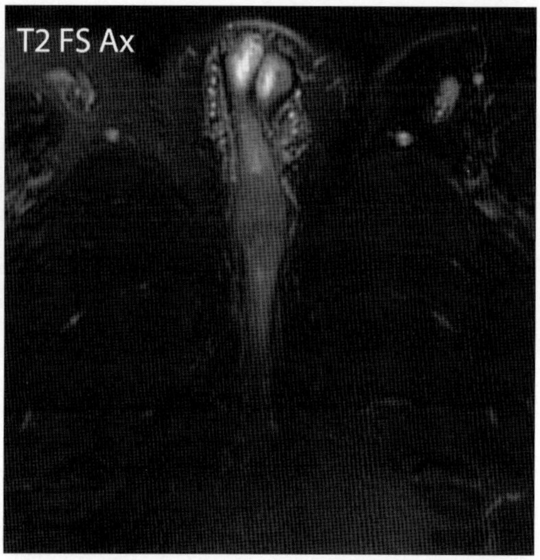

T2 FS Ax

Figure 90.2

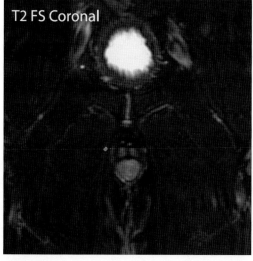

Figure 90.3

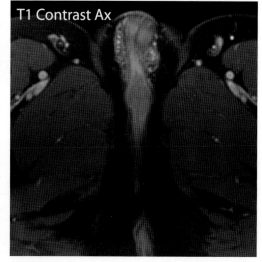

Figure 90.4

Case 90   Penile Cancer

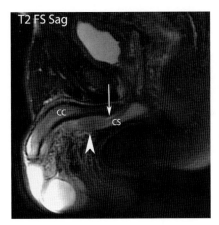

Figure 90.5

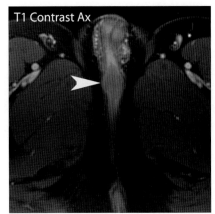

Figure 90.6

Findings

▶ Sagittal, axial, and coronal fat-suppressed T2-weighted (Figures 90.1–90.3) and axial contrast-enhanced (Figure 90.4) MR images of the penis are shown. A mildly T2 hypointense enhancing lesion (arrowhead in Figures 90.5 and 90.6) is noted in the penile shaft. On the sagittal view Figure 90.5, the lesion involves the corpus spongiosum (CS) and urethra (arrow). The corpus cavernosum (CC) and tunica albuginea are not involved.

Differential Diagnosis

▶ Diagnosis of penile cancer is established by physical examination and biopsy. MR imaging is used for local staging. T1 tumor is limited to subepithelial tissue, T2 tumor invades the corpora, T3 tumor involves the urethra or prostate, and T4 tumor invades other adjacent structures. In this patient, the enhancing tumor involves not only the corpus spongiosum but also the urethra, which is consistent with T3 stage.

Teaching Points

▶ Penile cancer occurs in the sixth and seventh decades.
▶ It is strongly associated with phimosis. Incidence is three times higher in uncircumcised males compared with circumcised males.
▶ Squamous cell carcinoma constitutes 95% of penile cancers.
▶ Location of tumor is in glans penis (48%), prepuce (21%), glans and prepuce (9%), coronal sulcus (6%), and shaft (2%).
▶ Local metastasis usually occurs to inguinal lymph nodes.
▶ Regional lymph node metastasis is the most important prognostic factor.
▶ Half of patients with enlarged inguinal lymph nodes have reactive lymphadenopathy.
▶ Distant metastases are uncommon at presentation.

Management

▶ Surgical resection or radiation

Further Reading
Singh AK, Gonzalez-Torrez P, Kaewlai R, Tabatabaei S, Harisinghani MG. Imaging of penile neoplasm. *Semin Ultrasound CT MR*. 2007;28(4):287–296.

Case 91

History

- 70-year-old female with vaginal bleeding

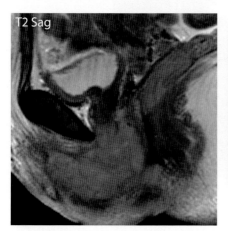

T2 Sag

Figure 91.1

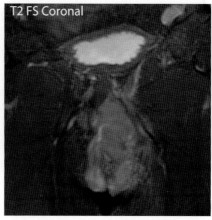

T2 FS Coronal

Figure 91.2

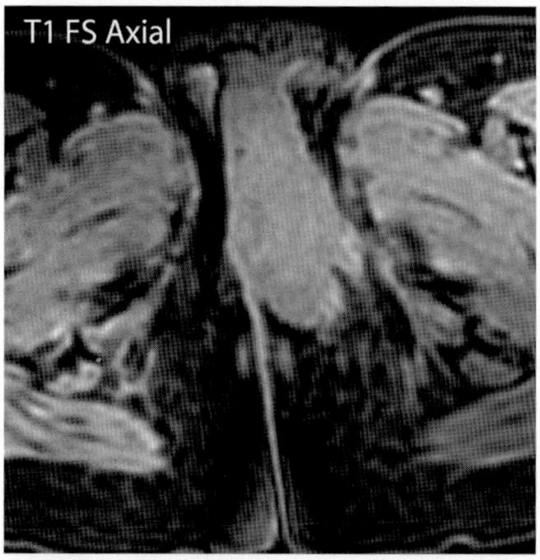

T1 FS Axial

Figure 91.3

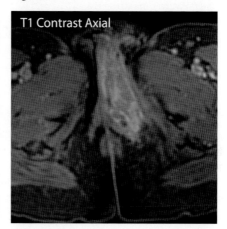

T1 Contrast Axial

Figure 91.4

T1 Contrast Sag

Figure 91.5

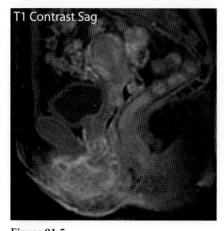

PET CT

Figure 91.6

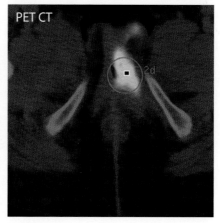

Case 91 Vulvar Carcinoma

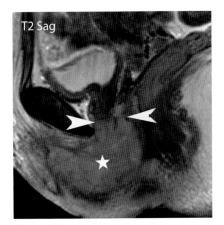

Figure 91.7

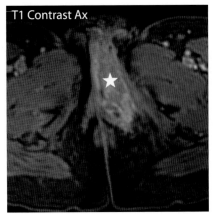

Figure 91.8

Findings

▶ Nonfat-suppressed sagittal (Figure 91.1) and fat-suppressed coronal (Figure 91.2) T2-weighted MR images show a large hyperintense vulvar mass (asterisk in 91.7 and 91.8) that involves the lower urethra and lower vagina (arrowheads) and extends into the perineal subcutaneous fat. Mass is isointense on T1 imaging (Figure 91.3) and shows heterogeneous enhancement (Figures 91.4 and 91.5). No groin lymphadenopathy is identified.

▶ The mass is strongly fludeoxyglucose (FDG) avid on positron emission tomography–computed tomography (PET–CT; Figure 91.6).

Differential Diagnosis

▶ The large infiltrating mass noted in this patient is consistent with a neoplastic process centered in the vulva with extension to the lower vagina and urethra. This pattern supports the diagnosis of primary vulvar carcinoma with secondary vaginal invasion over primary vaginal carcinoma. Primary vaginal malignancy is rare; secondary vaginal involvement by vulvar, cervical, or anorectal malignancy is more common. The diagnosis of squamous cell carcinoma of the vulva was established by biopsy in this patient.

Teaching Points

▶ Vulvar carcinoma constitutes 3%–5% of female genitourinary tract malignancy.

▶ The majority occur in women aged >70 years.

▶ Squamous cell carcinoma constitutes 85% of vulvar carcinomas. Melanoma and lymphoma are other uncommon vulvar malignancies.

▶ MRI is used to delineate local extension into the urethra, vagina, and anorectum for surgical planning as well as identification of lymph nodal spread.

▶ Lymphatic spread occurs in inguinal/femoral lymph nodes and indicates worse prognosis.

▶ Patients without groin node involvement have 90% survival versus 50% survival of patients with groin node involvement.

▶ FDG PET–CT can be used to assess lymph nodal involvement, extranodal disease, and treatment response.

Management

▶ Surgical excision and/or radiotherapy

Further Reading

Griffin N, Grant LA, Sala E. Magnetic resonance imaging of vaginal and vulval pathology. *Eur Radiol.* 2008;18(6):1269–1280.

Section VII

Testis, Epididymis, and Scrotum

History

► 33-year-old male with palpable testicular mass

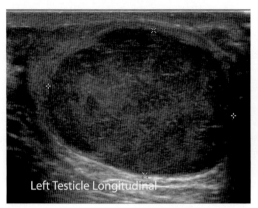

Figure 92.1

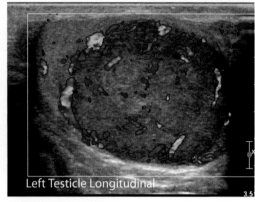

Figure 92.2

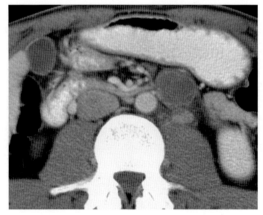

Figure 92.3

Case 92 Testicular Cancer

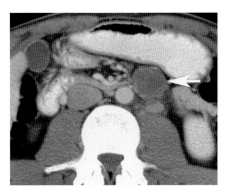

Figure 92.4

Findings

▸ Grayscale and Doppler ultrasound images of the left testicle (Figures 92.1 and 92.2) show a large, well-defined, hypoechoic solid vascular mass replacing most of the left testicle.

▸ Contrast-enhanced CT image (Figure 92.3) shows left para-aortic retroperitoneal lymphadenopathy (arrow in Figure 92.4).

Differential Diagnosis

▸ Differential diagnosis of a solid testicular mass includes primary testicular cancer, lymphoma, epidermoid cyst, and granulomatous disease. Testicular cancer and lymphoma can have similar imaging appearance, but lymphoma is less likely in this case as it is more often multifocal or diffuse and occurs in an older age group. Granulomatous orchitis due to fungal or tubercular infection usually has concomitant epididymitis. Testicular sarcoid is commonly bilateral and multifocal. Epidermoid cysts are well-defined benign lesions with calcifications and a typical whorled appearance. Germ cell cancer is the most common solid testicular mass in a young patient. The diagnosis of seminoma was confirmed on histopathology. Presence of enlarged periaortic lymph nodes is consistent with regional metastatic lymphadenopathy.

Teaching Points

▸ Germ cell tumors are almost always malignant and constitute 95% of primary testicular neoplasms. Seminoma is the most common type of germ cell tumor. Embryonal carcinoma, yolk sac tumor, choriocarcinoma, teratoma, and mixed tumors constitute the rest.

▸ Sex cord (Sertoli cell) and stromal (Leydig cell) tumors are non-germ cell testicular neoplasms that are usually benign.

▸ Peak incidence is in those aged 20–40 years.

▸ Testicular cancer is rare in blacks, and sarcoidosis should be considered in the differential for testicular lesions in the black population.

▸ Risk factors include prior testicular tumor, cryptorchidism, infertility, family history, and intersex syndromes.

▸ Testicular germ cell tumors (except choriocarcinoma) have lymphatic spread along testicular veins to the para-aortic lymph nodes.

▸ Regional metastatic lymphadenopathy is ipsilateral to the tumor. Left testicular tumors initially metastasize to the left periaortic lymph nodes and right-sided tumors to the aortocaval nodes.

Management

▸ Orchiectomy with radiation and/or chemotherapy

Further Reading

Woodward PJ, Sohaey R, O'Donoghue MJ, Green DE. From the archives of the AFIP: tumors and tumorlike lesions of the testis: radiologic-pathologic correlation. *Radiographics*. 2002;22(1):189–216.

History

▸ 60-year-old male with scrotal mass and malaise

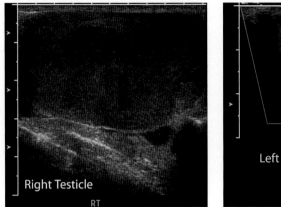

Figure 93.1

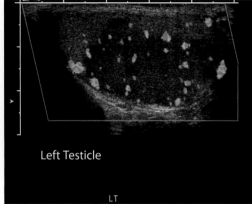

Figure 93.2

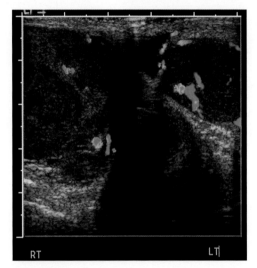

Figure 93.3

Case 93   Testicular Lymphoma

Findings

▶ Grayscale and color Doppler images of both testicles (Figures 93.1–93.3) reveal large bilateral ill-defined hypoechoic lesions replacing most of the testicular parenchyma. The lesions have increased vascularity compared with the uninvolved parenchyma.

Differential Diagnosis

▶ Differential diagnosis of bilateral testicular masses includes germ cell tumors (seminoma being most common), lymphoma, and sarcoid. Lymphoma and seminoma both have similar imaging appearance, but older age and bilaterality favor the diagnosis of lymphoma in this patient. Seminoma commonly occurs in a younger (aged 20–35 years) population. Sarcoid often has concomitant involvement of the testicle and epididymis. The diagnosis of lymphoma was confirmed on orchiectomy.

Teaching Points

▶ Primary lymphoma of the testis constitutes 1%–9% of all testicular tumors.

▶ Lymphoma is the most common testicular tumor in those aged >60 years.

▶ Lymphoma appears as diffuse or focal areas of decreased echogenicity, with maintenance of the testicular ovoid shape.

▶ Testicular lymphoma lesions are usually hypervascular on color Doppler.

▶ Local spread to the epididymis, spermatic cord, and skin can occur.

▶ Bilateral testicular involvement is seen in 35% of patients.

Management

▶ Orchiectomy followed by chemotherapy

Further Reading

Mazzu D, Jeffrey RB Jr, Ralls PW. Lymphoma and leukemia involving the testicles: findings on gray-scale and color Doppler sonography. *AJR Am J Roentgenol.* 1995;164(3):645–647.

History

▶ 35-year-old man presents with acute right testicular pain

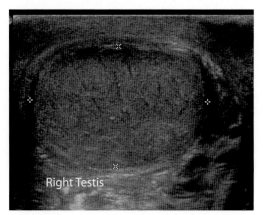

Figure 94.1

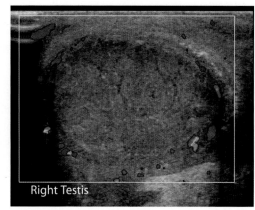

Figure 94.2

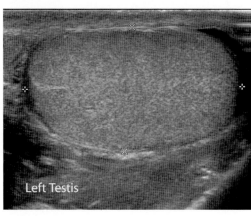

Figure 94.3

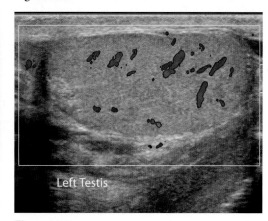

Figure 94.4

Case 94 Testicular Torsion

Findings

▶ Grayscale image of the right testicle (Figure 94.1) shows heterogeneous decreased testicular echotexture with scrotal wall thickening. Color Doppler image of the right testis (Figure 94.2) shows absent intratesticular flow with peripheral vascularity around the testis.

▶ Grayscale and color Doppler images of the contralateral left testis (Figures 94.3 and 94.4) show normal homogeneous echotexture with maintained intratesticular vascularity.

Differential Diagnosis

▶ Differential diagnosis of acute unilateral scrotal pain includes epididymo-orchitis, testicular torsion, and torsion of testicular appendage. Epididymo-orchitis and testicular torsion can both cause decreased heterogeneous testicular echotexture. Epididymo-orchitis causes increased testicular and epididymal vascularity. The absence of testicular vascularity noted here is diagnostic of testicular torsion. Torsion of testicular appendage is seen in adolescents. The torsed appendage is identified as a hyperechoic structure adjacent to a normal-appearing testis or epididymis.

Teaching Points

▶ Testicular torsion is a surgical emergency caused by twisting of the spermatic cord compromising testicular blood flow.

▶ Bell clapper deformity (tunica vaginalis insertion high in the spermatic cord) allows increased mobility of testis and predisposes to torsion.

▶ It presents with sudden onset of scrotal pain, swelling, and redness.

▶ Absence of intratesticular flow on Doppler is the most important imaging feature and is 100% specific, 86% sensitive, and 97% accurate for torsion in painful scrotum.

▶ Normal testicular echotexture may be present in early torsion (1–3 hours). Edema and decreased echotexture are seen in 4–6 hours. Heterogeneous echotexture develops by 24 hours due to infarction, congestion, and hemorrhage.

▶ An abrupt change in size and shape of the spermatic cord at the external inguinal ring indicates location of the twist.

▶ Torsion may be complete, incomplete, or transient.

▶ Normal testicular echotexture is a good indicator of testicular viability.

Management

▶ Emergent surgical detorsion if detected early

Further Reading
Dogra VS, Gottlieb RH, Oka M, Rubens DJ. Sonography of the scrotum. *Radiology*. 2003;227(1):18–36.

History

► 23-year-old male with injury to the scrotum

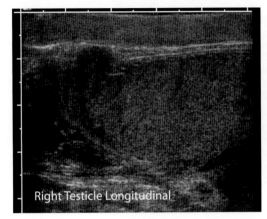

Figure 95.1

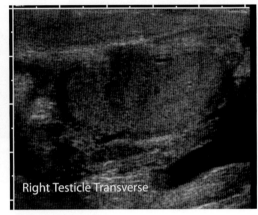

Figure 95.2

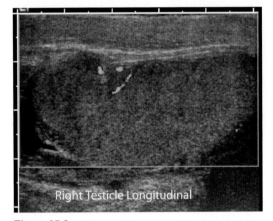

Figure 95.3

Case 95   Testicular Rupture

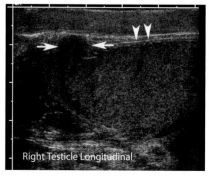

Right Testicle Longitudinal

Figure 95.4

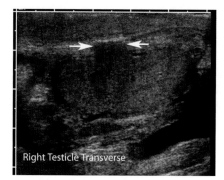

Right Testicle Transverse

Figure 95.5

Findings

▶ Longitudinal and transverse ultrasound images of right testicle (Figures 95.1 and 95.2) show focal disruption of tunica albuginea with contour deformity and extrusion of testicular parenchyma (arrows in Figures 95.4 and 95.5). Focal heterogeneity is present within the testicle adjacent to the tunica discontinuity. Arrowheads in Figure 95.4 identify the normal hyperechoic tunica albuginea.

▶ Doppler image (Figure 95.3) shows decreased vascularity in the extruded part of the parenchyma with normal adjacent vascularity.

Differential Diagnosis

▶ In a patient with testicular trauma, after identifying the presence of testicular injury, the goal of imaging is to differentiate testicular rupture from lesser injuries that can cause intratesticular hematomas with intact tunica. In this patient, identification of testicular contour deformity with parenchymal heterogeneity is highly specific for testicular rupture. Direct visualization of the breach in tunica further confirms the diagnosis. Intratesticular hematomas cause parenchymal heterogeneity but do not show contour deformity or tunica breach.

Teaching Points

▶ Encapsulation of the testicles by tunica albuginea, laxity of scrotal skin, and cremasteric reflex protect the testicles from trauma.

▶ Testicular rupture is caused by disruption of the tunica albuginea. Its identification is of paramount importance as surgical repair within 72 hours of injury can salvage about 80% of ruptured testicles. On the other hand, intratesticular hematoma is treated conservatively.

▶ Ultrasound can be extremely sensitive (up to 100%) and specific (65%–93%) in detecting rupture.

▶ Contour deformity due to extrusion of testicular parenchyma in combination with heterogeneous parenchymal echotexture is highly suggestive of testicular rupture.

▶ Tunica albuginea is identified as two parallel hyperechoic lines outlining the testis. Focal discontinuity of tunica is characteristic of rupture; if used alone, it will result in low sensitivity (50%) and a high false-negative rate.

▶ Absence of vascularity on Doppler is concerning for devascularized testicular parenchyma that requires debridement.

Management

▶ Immediate surgical repair

Further Reading

Guichard G, El Ammari J, Del Coro C, et al. Accuracy of ultrasonography in diagnosis of testicular rupture after blunt scrotal trauma. *Urology.* 2008;71(1):52–56.

History

▶ 35-year-old male with scrotal discomfort

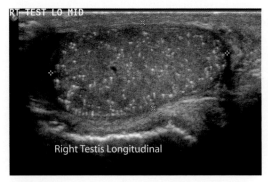

Figure 96.1

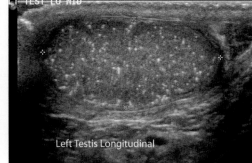

Figure 96.2

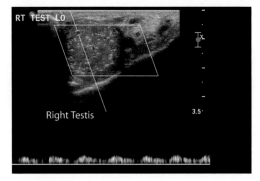

Figure 96.3

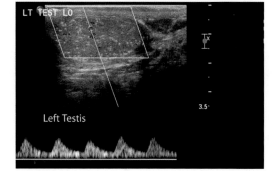

Figure 96.4

Case 96 Testicular Microlithiasis

Findings

▶ Grayscale ultrasound images of both testicles (Figures 96.1 and 96.2) reveal innumerable tiny, nonshadowing echogenic foci throughout both testicles. No discrete testicular mass is identified.

▶ Color Doppler images of both testicles (Figures 96.3 and 96.4) show normal testicular blood flow.

Differential Diagnosis

▶ A small number of scattered echogenic foci in the testicles is considered limited testicular microlithiasis, while the presence of more than five foci per transducer field (innumerable foci in this case) is consistent with classic testicular microlithiasis. Lack of acoustic shadowing is also typical of microlithiasis and helps differentiate it from other causes of testicular calcifications.

Teaching Points

▶ Classic testicular microlithiasis is defined as the presence of five or more microliths in either or both testicles on at least one ultrasound image.

▶ It is an uncommon incidental finding on testicular ultrasound.

▶ Echogenic foci likely represent tiny calcifications within tubules.

▶ Testicular microlithiasis has been associated with testicular malignancy, but it is controversial whether it is an independent risk factor for malignancy.

▶ Follow-up is recommended due to its association with malignancy.

▶ Physical examination, self-examination, or ultrasound can be used for follow-up. No consensus exists on the type, duration, or interval of follow-up.

Management

▶ Follow-up with physical examination, self-examination, or ultrasound

Further Reading

Meissner A, Mamoulakis C, de la Rosette JJ, Pes MP. Clinical update on testicular microlithiasis. *Curr Opin Urol.* 2009;19(6):615–618.

Case 97

History

- 27-year-old male with palpable scrotal lump

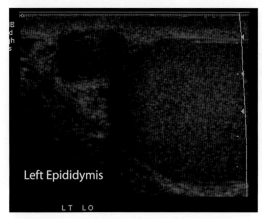

Figure 97.1

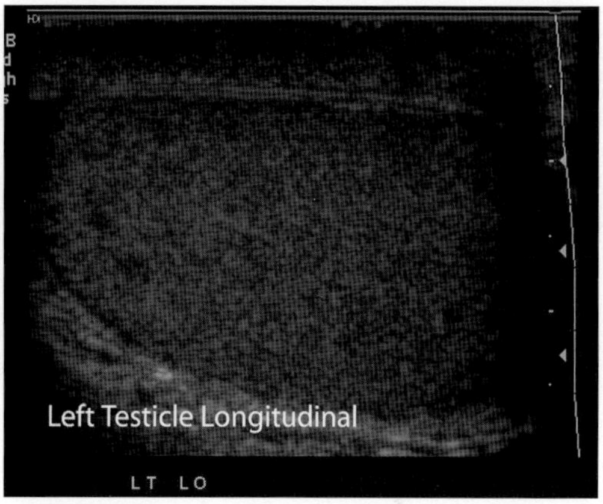

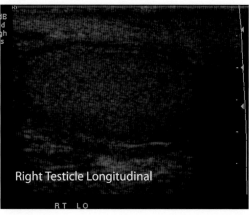

Figure 97.2

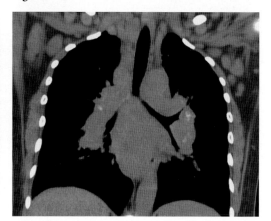

Figure 97.3

Figure 97.4

Case 97 Testicular Sarcoid

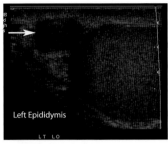

Figure 97.5

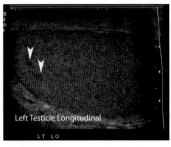

Figure 97.6

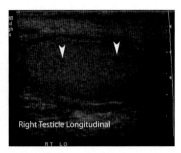

Figure 97.7

Findings

▶ Grayscale ultrasound image of the left epididymis (Figure 97.1) reveals a well-defined hypoechoic solid left epididymal nodule (arrow in Figure 97.5).

▶ Longitudinal grayscale images of the left and right testicle (Figures 97.2 and 97.3) show small bilateral hypoechoic nodules (arrowheads in Figures 97.6 and 97.7).

▶ Coronal CT reconstruction of the chest (Figure 97.4) shows extensive bilateral hilar, mediastinal, axillary, and supraclavicular lymphadenopathy with calcifications.

Differential Diagnosis

▶ Solid testicular lesions raise concern for malignant processes such as germ cell tumors or lymphoma. Solid epididymal masses are uncommon and usually represent benign adenomatoid tumors. The presence of concomitant epididymal and testicular nodules would be an unusual presentation for malignancy but is a common feature of genitourinary sarcoidosis. The presence of extensive calcifying lymphadenopathy in the chest is also consistent with sarcoidosis.

Teaching Points

▶ Sarcoidosis is a multisystem granulomatous disease that affects various organ systems.

▶ Genitourinary sarcoidosis is uncommon and occurs in 5% of patients with sarcoidosis in autopsy series.

▶ The epididymis is the most common site of reproductive tract involvement and is involved in 70% of cases followed by testes in 47%.

▶ Testicular sarcoid has a preponderance in black males aged 20–40 years.

▶ Testicular involvement is often associated with epididymal disease, but there may be isolated testicular involvement.

▶ Clinical presentation is with painless palpable scrotal mass.

▶ On imaging, testicular sarcoid usually presents as small bilateral solid lesions.

▶ Sarcoid lesions usually respond to steroid treatment.

▶ Correct identification of testicular sarcoid is important in order to avoid unnecessary orchiectomy.

Management

▶ Antiinflammatory drugs

Further Reading

Woodward PJ, Sohaey R, O'Donoghue MJ, Green DE. From the archives of the AFIP: tumors and tumorlike lesions of the testis: radiologic-pathologic correlation. *Radiographics*. 2002;22(1):189–216.

History

▶ 55-year-old male with scrotal lump

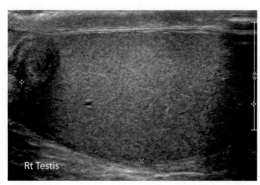

Figure 98.1

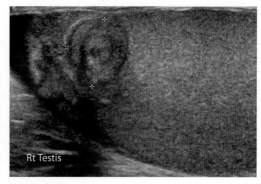

Figure 98.2

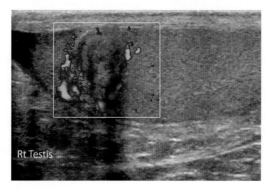

Figure 98.3

Case 98 Testicular Adenomatoid Tumor

Findings

▶ Grayscale and color Doppler images of the left testicle (Figures 98.1–98.3) show a well-defined solid heterogeneous nodule in the periphery of the testis (calipers) that abuts the adjacent epididymal head. The lesion does not show significant vascularity.

Differential Diagnosis

▶ A peripherally located solid testicular neoplasm such as germ cell tumor (younger population) or lymphoma (in the elderly) and granulomatous conditions such as sarcoid are included in the differential diagnosis. However, careful evaluation of the images suggests that the lesion may be centered in the tunica albuginea (and not the testicular parenchyma) with indentation/extension into the testicular parenchyma and epididymis. This raises the possibility of a benign adenomatoid tumor arising from the tunica albuginea. Although a tunical origin was suspected, it was not possible to confidently exclude a peripheral testicular tumor on the basis of imaging. Surgical excision was performed to confirm the diagnosis of an adenomatoid tumor of the testicular tunica.

Teaching Points

▶ Adenomatoid tumors are the most common paratesticular neoplasm.
▶ Adenomatoid tumors are benign tumors of mesothelial origin.
▶ Adenomatoid tumors commonly arise from the epididymis. However, about 14% arise from the testicular tunica.
▶ Differentiation of solid intratesticular tumors from paratesticular tumors is important, as the former are usually malignant while the latter are benign.

Management

▶ Local surgical excision

Further Reading

Mäkäräinen HP, Tammela TL, Karttunen TJ, Mattila SI, Hellström PA, Kontturi MJ. Intrascrotal adenomatoid tumors and their ultrasound findings. *J Clin Ultrasound*. 1993;21(1):33–37.

History

► 58-year-old male with scrotal mass

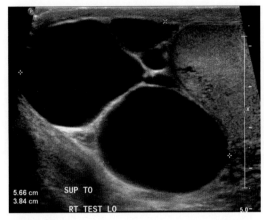

Figure 99.1

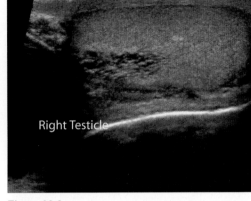

Figure 99.2

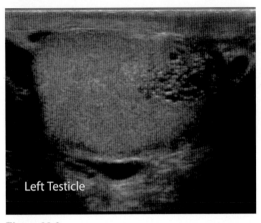

Figure 99.3

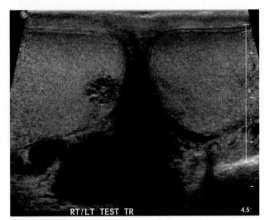

Figure 99.4

Case 99   Epididymal Cyst with Tubular Ectasia of Rete Testis

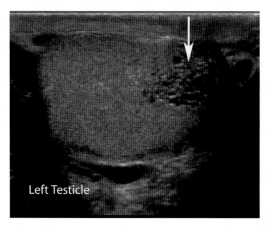

Left Testicle

Figure 99.5

Findings

▶ Ultrasound image (Figure 99.1) reveals a large multiloculated cystic structure superior to the right testicle in the expected region of the epididymal head (calipers).

▶ Focal aggregation of numerous tiny cystic tubular structures is noted in both testicles (Figures 99.2–99.4, arrow in Figure 99.5).

Differential Diagnosis

▶ Differential diagnosis of cystic lesions in the epididymal head includes spermatocele and true epididymal cyst. Spermatoceles and epididymal cysts are indistinguishable on imaging and appear as anechoic unilocular or multilocular cystic structures adjacent to the testicle. Either of these can cause seminiferous tubule obstruction and lead to tubular ectasia of rete testis (cystic rete). The bilateral focal aggregation of tiny dilated tubular structures along the mediastinum testis noted here represents tubular ectasia of rete testis, likely due to obstruction caused by the large epididymal cyst.

Teaching Points

▶ Cystic lesions in the epididymal head are present in 20%–40% of the asymptomatic population.

▶ True epididymal head cysts are lymphatic in origin and contain clear fluid.

▶ Spermatoceles are caused by obstruction of the ductal system and have milky contents with cellular debris and spermatozoa.

▶ Epididymal cystadenomas are rare epididymal cystic tumors seen in patients with von Hippel–Lindau syndrome.

▶ Rete testes are irregular anastomosing spaces formed as the seminiferous tubules enter the mediastinum testis and lead to efferent ducts and epididymis.

▶ Tubular ectasia of rete testis is a benign condition.

▶ On ultrasound, tiny cystic spaces without solid component in periphery of mediastinum testis are pathognomic of tubular ectasia of rete testis.

▶ Most patients with tubular ectasia of rete testis have an underlying cause of ductal obstruction such as epididymal cyst/spermatocele, prior vasectomy, or inguinal hernia repair.

▶ Lack of color flow in tubular ectasia differentiates it from cystic testicular neoplasm (rare).

Management

▶ If asymptomatic, treatment is not necessary. Chronic pain may require epididymectomy.

Further Reading
Burrus JK, Lockhart ME, Kenney PJ, Kolettis PN. Cystic ectasia of the rete testis: clinical and radiographic features. *J Urol.* 2002;168(4 Pt 1):1436–1438.

Case 100

History

- 34-year-old man with acute right scrotal pain

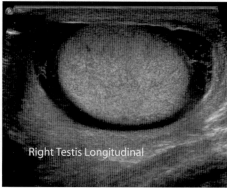

Figure 100.1

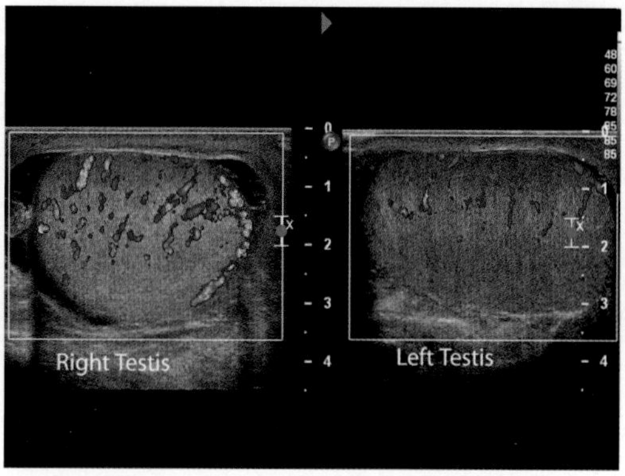

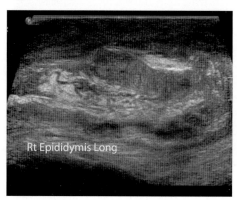

Figure 100.2

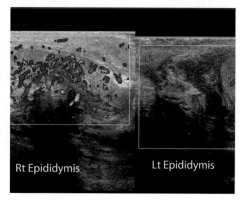

Figure 100.3

Figure 100.4

Case 100 Epididymo-orchitis with Pyocele

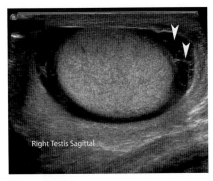

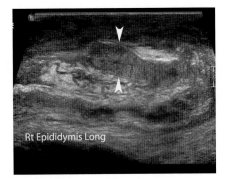

Figure 100.5 **Figure 100.6**

Findings

▶ Sagittal grayscale image of the right testicle (Figure 100.1) reveals a normal-appearing right testicle. A moderate amount of fluid with internal septations surrounds the testicle (arrowheads in Figure 100.5).

▶ Color Doppler side-by-side image of both testicles (Figure 100.2) shows markedly increased right testicular vascularity compared with the left testicle.

▶ Grayscale image of the right epididymis (Figure 100.3) reveals a markedly enlarged right epididymis (arrowheads in Figure 100.6).

▶ Color Doppler side-by-side image of epididymis shows enlargement and increased vascularity of the right epididymis when compared with the normal-appearing left epididymis (Figure 100.4).

Differential Diagnosis

▶ It is clinically difficult to differentiate epididymitis/epididymo-orchitis from testicular torsion; on ultrasound, these entities have different appearances. Torsion has decreased testicular vascularity, while the enlargement and hyperemia of the epididymis seen in this patient is typical of epididymitis. Increased vascularity of the right testicle, which is present in this patient, suggests associated orchitis. The septated fluid around the right testicle is consistent with a pyocele.

Teaching Points

▶ Epididymitis is the most common cause of acute scrotal pain.

▶ The source of infection is usually in the lower urinary tract (urethra, prostate, bladder) and reaches the epididymis through the vas deferens.

▶ Orchitis is present in 20% of patients with epididymitis.

▶ On ultrasound, early epididymitis/epididymo-orchitis is identified by increased vascularity on the symptomatic side. This may be present before grayscale changes of decreased epididymal/testicular echotexture and increased epididymal size.

▶ Pyocele and abscess formation are potential complications.

Management

▶ Antibiotics

Further Reading
Lee JC, Bhatt S, Dogra VS. Imaging of the epididymis. *Ultrasound Q.* 2008;24(1):3–16.

History

▶ 63-year-old man with scrotal pain, swelling, and crepitus

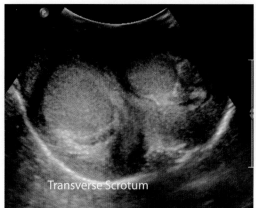

Figure 101.1

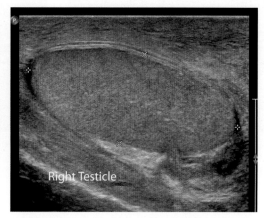

Figure 101.2

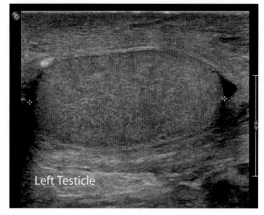

Figure 101.3

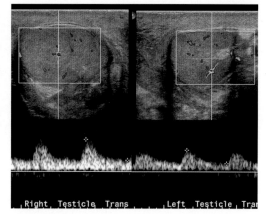

Figure 101.4

Case 101 Fournier's Gangrene

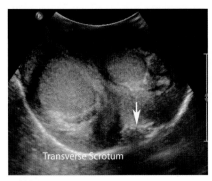

Figure 101.5

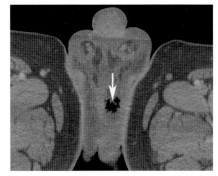

Figure 101.6

Findings

▶ Grayscale transverse ultrasound image of the scrotum (Figure 101.1) shows severe scrotal wall edema. An echogenic focus with dirty shadowing is present in the scrotal wall (arrow in Figure 101.5).

▶ Grayscale and color Doppler images (Figures 101.2–101.4) of both testicles show normal testicular echotexture and vascularity.

▶ Axial CT image (Figure 101.6) reveals extensive scrotal fat stranding with a focus of gas within the soft tissues (arrow).

Differential Diagnosis

▶ Differential diagnosis of acute scrotal pain and swelling includes epididymo-orchitis, testicular torsion, incarcerated inguinal hernia, cellulitis, and Fournier's gangrene. Normal testicular echotexture and vascularity in this patient exclude epididymo-orchitis and torsion, while absence of bowel loops in the scrotum rules out an incarcerated hernia. Scrotal wall thickening, as seen here, can be present in cellulitis as well as Fournier's gangrene. Presence of echogenic focus with dirty shadowing in the scrotal wall indicates a pocket of gas, consistent with the diagnosis of Fournier's gangrene

Teaching Points

▶ Fournier's gangrene is a rapidly progressing polymicrobial necrotizing fasciitis of the perineum.

▶ It is a urologic emergency with mortality ranging from 15%–50%.

▶ Diabetes and alcoholism are common predisposing factors.

▶ Most patients have an underlying source of infection that may be colorectal, urologic, or cutaneous. Ten percent of cases are idiopathic.

▶ Presentation is with sudden onset perineal pain, swelling, crepitus, redness, fever, and leukocytosis.

▶ Rapid spread of infection causes obliterative endarteritis, resulting in necrosis along superficial and deep fascial planes.

▶ On imaging, subcutaneous scrotal gas is pathognomic of Fournier's gangrene.

▶ Fournier's gangrene is a clinical diagnosis, but CT demonstrates the extent of subcutaneous gas and inflammation and often identifies the source of infection.

Management

▶ Immediate complete surgical debridement of necrotic tissue and intravenous antibiotics

Further Reading
Levenson RB, Singh AK, Novelline RA. Fournier gangrene: role of imaging. *Radiographics*. 2008;28(2):519–528.

History

▶ 31-year-old man with infertility

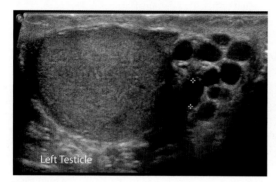

Figure 102.1

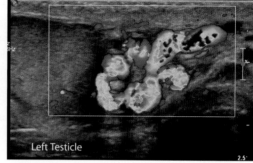

Figure 102.2

Case 102 Varicocele

Findings

► Grayscale and color Doppler images of the left scrotum (Figures 102.1 and 102.2) show multiple, dilated, hypoechoic, tubular structures adjacent and superior to the left testicle that demonstrate color flow.

Differential Diagnosis

► Hypoechoic, serpiginous vascular structures represent dilated veins of the pampniform plexus. Veins of the pampniform plexus are adjacent to the testicles and normally measure approximately 1–1.5 mm. Dilation of the veins >3 mm with (or without) Valsalva maneuver is considered diagnostic of a varicocele.

Teaching Points

► Most varicoceles are idiopathic (or primary) and occur due to incompetent valves in the gonadal veins.
► Primary varicoceles usually occur at the age of 15–25 years and are present in 15% of all males.
► On physical examination, varicoceles feel like a "bag of worms."
► Unilateral varicoceles are usually on the left (due to the long left testicular vein and its entry into the renal vein at a right angle).
► Secondary varicoceles develop due to increased pressure on gonadal vein secondary to compressing by retroperitoneal tumors, cirrhosis and portal hypertension.
► Unilateral right varicoceles should raise suspicion of a retroperitoneal mass obstructing the right gonadal vein.
► Clinical varicoceles have been implicated as a cause of male infertility and are associated with decreased sperm count.
► Subclinical varicoceles (identified on imaging but not on physical examination) do not have an established association with infertility and are usually not treated.
► Doppler ultrasound has a very high sensitivity for varicocele. Scanning with the patient standing increases sensitivity.
► Valsalva maneuver during ultrasound demonstrates increase in size of the dilated veins with increase in intraabdominal pressure.

Management

► Surgical excision or embolization

Further Reading
Dogra VS, Gottlieb RH, Oka M, Rubens DJ. Sonography of the scrotum. *Radiology*. 2003;227(1):18–36.

Section VIII Uterus and Fallopian Tube

History

▶ 43-year-old female with pelvic pain

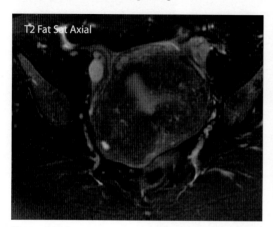

Figure 103.1

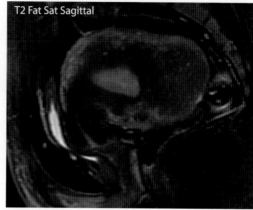

Figure 103.2

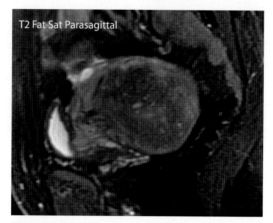

Figure 103.3

Case 103 Uterine Adenomyosis

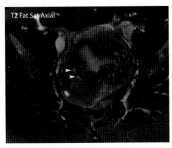
Figure 103.4

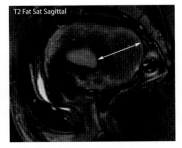
Figure 103.5

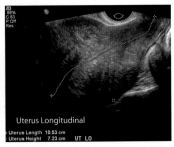
Figure 103.6

Findings

▶ Axial, sagittal, and parasagittal fat-suppressed T2-weighted images (Figures 103.1–103.3) show an enlarged uterus with diffuse as well as focal thickening of the T2 hypointense junctional zone (double-headed arrow in Figure 103.5). Tiny T2 hyperintense cystic foci (arrowheads in Figure 103.4) are scattered throughout the thickened junctional zone.

▶ Figure 103.6 from a different patient shows a heterogeneous enlarged uterus on ultrasound.

Differential Diagnosis

▶ The junctional zone is the T2 hypointense layer between the hyperintense endometrium and intermediate signal myometrium. Focal or diffuse thickening of the junctional zone >12 mm (as noted here) is suggestive of adenomyosis. Tiny T2 hyperintense cysts in the thickened junctional zone are also a feature of adenomyosis. Uterine fibroids have similar presentation but are well demarcated, round T2 hypointense lesions that cause mass effect, which helps to differentiate them from the more ill-defined T2 hypointense thickening of the junctional zone with minimal mass effect seen in adenomyosis.

▶ On ultrasound, adenomyosis presents as an enlarged, diffusely heterogeneous uterus, as seen in Figure 103.6.

Teaching Points

▶ Adenomyosis is caused by the penetration of endometrial glands into the myometrium adjacent to the endometrium.

▶ It may be "diffuse" and include the entire endometrial myometrial interface or be "focal" and limited to an area.

▶ Adenomyosis is a common benign disease and often presents with dysmenorrhea and menorrhagia in perimenopausal women.

▶ Uterine fibroids are present in 36%–50% of adenomyosis cases.

▶ On MRI, junctional zone thickening >12 mm has a diagnostic accuracy of 85% and specificity of 96% for adenomyosis.

▶ Identification of tiny T2 hyperintense microcysts within the junctional zone is pathognomonic of adenomyosis but seen in only half of cases.

▶ An adenomyoma is a rare focal collection of abnormal endometrial glands in the myometrium separate from the junctional zone.

Management

▶ Hysterectomy for severe disease

Further Reading

Novellas S, Chassang M, Delotte J, et al. MRI characteristics of the uterine junctional zone: from normal to the diagnosis of adenomyosis. *AJR Am J Roentgenol.* 2011;196(5):1206–1213.

History

▶ 38-year-old female with menorrhagia

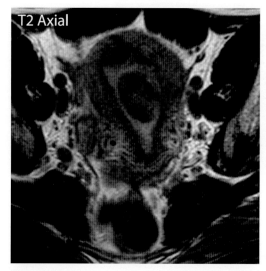

Figure 104.1

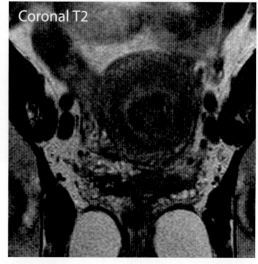

Figure 104.2

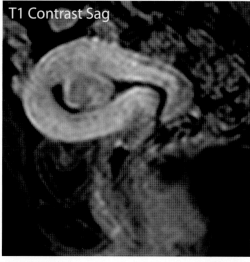

Figure 104.3

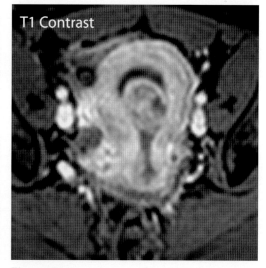

Figure 104.4

Case 104 Submucosal Uterine Fibroid

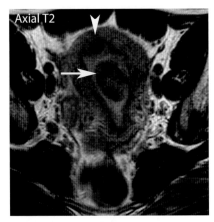

Figure 104.5

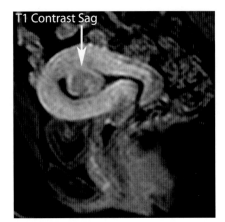

Figure 104.6

Findings

▶ Axial and coronal T2-weighted images through the pelvis (Figures 104.1 and 104.2) show a well-defined, T2 hypointense, intracavitary lesion that expands the endometrial cavity (arrow in Figure 104.5). A small T2 hypointense fibroid is present in the fundal myometrium (arrowhead in Figure 104.5). A small amount of endometrial fluid is present.

▶ Contrast-enhanced sagittal and axial fat-suppressed T1-weighted images (Figures 104.3 and 104.4) show enhancement of the intracavitary lesion. The sagittal image demonstrates its attachment to the myometrium (arrow in Figure 104.6).

Differential Diagnosis

▶ Differential diagnosis of an intracavitary uterine lesion includes endometrial hyperplasia, endometrial carcinoma, endometrial polyp, and submucosal fibroid. Endometrial carcinoma and hyperplasia cause diffuse endometrial involvement with a broad base of attachment and can be excluded here. Endometrial polyps and submucosal fibroids appear as well-defined intracavitary lesions. Polyps are usually T2 hyperintense and have a narrow stalk. Submucosal fibroids are T2 hypointense and usually have a wider attachment. The low T2 signal intensity (similar to the fundal fibroid) and wide attachment to the endometrium favor the diagnosis of a submucosal fibroid in this patient.

Teaching Points

▶ Fibroids or leiomyomas are common benign tumors of smooth muscle that occur in 1 in 5 women aged >30 years.
▶ Intramural fibroids grow within the myometrium; subserosal fibroids grow under the serosa, distorting the outer uterine contour; and submucosal fibroids grow under the submucosa, projecting into the endometrial cavity.
▶ Fibroids (especially submucosal fibroids) are a common cause of menorrhagia, dysmenorrhea, and infertility.
▶ On ultrasound, submucosal fibroids have overlying echogenic endometrium that helps to differentiate them from endometrial polyps, which arise from the endometrium.
▶ Submucosal fibroids that project more than 50% into the uterine cavity can be removed by hysteroscopic myomectomy.
▶ Submucosal fibroids can become intracavitary after uterine artery embolization, but the majority are spontaneously expelled without symptoms.

Management

▶ Myomectomy or uterine artery embolization

Further Reading

Deshmukh SP, Gonsalves CF, Guglielmo FF, Mitchell DG. Role of MR imaging of uterine leiomyomas before and after embolization. *Radiographics.* 2012;32(6):E251–281.

History

▶ 35-year-old female with vaginal bleeding

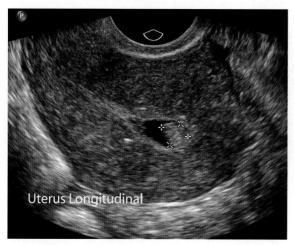

Figure 105.1

Case 105 Endometrial Polyp

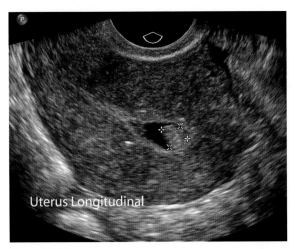

Figure 105.2

Findings

▶ Longitudinal ultrasound image of the uterus (Figures 105.1 and 105.2) shows a small echogenic nodular lesion in the endometrial cavity (calipers) outlined by endometrial fluid. The lesion is isoechoic to the endometrium.

Differential Diagnosis

▶ Differential diagnosis of focal endometrial thickening includes endometrial polyp, endometrial hyperplasia, endometrial carcinoma, and submucosal fibroid. Endometrial carcinoma and hyperplasia cause diffuse endometrial thickening with a broad base rather than focal thickening. Submucosal fibroids and polyps are both well-defined endometrial lesions, with polyps having a narrow attachment or stalk and fibroids having a broad attachment. Polyps appear to arise from the endometrium and are often isoechoic to the echogenic endometrium. On the contrary, submucosal fibroids have overlying echogenic endometrium. In this patient, the well-defined echogenic polypoid lesion delineated by endometrial fluid appears to arise from the endometrium and is consistent with a polyp.

Teaching Points

▶ Endometrial polyps commonly present with vaginal bleeding.
▶ It is noted that 95.2% of endometrial polyps are benign. Older menopausal women with bleeding have a higher risk of malignancy.
▶ Endometrial polyps may be associated with infertility.
▶ Tamoxifen therapy is associated with endometrial polyps.
▶ Imaging appearance overlaps with submucosal fibroid.
▶ An endometrial polyp appears as an echogenic filling defect in the endometrial cavity or focal endometrial thickening. A vascular stalk may be seen.
▶ Most polyps are homogeneously hyperechoic, but cystic foci may be present.
▶ Sonohysterography or transvaginal ultrasound performed during instillation of saline into the endometrial cavity allows improved visualization of endometrial polyps.

Management

▶ Polypectomy in symptomatic or postmenopausal women

Further Reading
Steinkeler JA, Woodfield CA, Lazarus E, Hillstrom MM. Female infertility: a systematic approach to radiologic imaging and diagnosis. *Radiographics*. 2009;29(5):1353–1370.

History

▶ 40-year-old woman with vaginal bleeding and positive pregnancy test

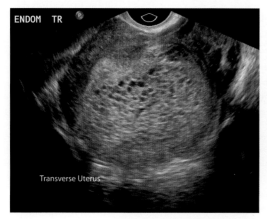

Figure 106.1

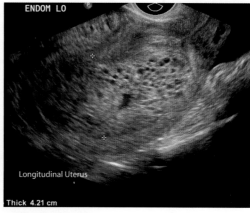

Figure 106.2

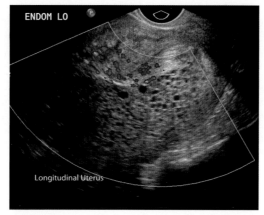

Figure 106.3

Case 106 Hydatiform Mole

Findings

▸ Grayscale transverse and longitudinal ultrasound images of the uterus (Figures 106.1 and 106.2) show a large echogenic lesion with innumerable cystic spaces filling up the uterine cavity. No definite myometrial involvement is identified. Color Doppler image (Figure 106.3) shows mild peripheral vascularity.

Differential Diagnosis

▸ In a patient with elevated human chorionic gonadotropin (HCG) level, the echogenic uterine lesion with numerous cystic spaces, as seen here, is diagnostic of a molar pregnancy. Lack of demonstrable fetal parts suggests a complete hydatiform mole. Absence of demonstrable myometrial invasion makes an invasive mole or choriocarcinoma less likely.

Teaching Points

▸ Gestational trophoblastic disease is a spectrum of disorders caused by abnormal proliferation of pregnancy-associated trophoblasts that range from hydatiform mole (complete or partial), to invasive mole, to choriocarcinoma. Lesions that invade locally or metastasize are also grouped together as gestational trophoblastic neoplasia.

▸ A complete hydatiform mole is the most common form of gestational trophoblastic disease.

▸ Molar pregnancy is common in women aged <20 years and >35 years.

▸ Fetal parts are absent in a complete hydatiform mole. An incomplete mole has associated fetal parts.

▸ Clinically, molar pregnancy presents with enlarged uterus, vaginal bleeding, and rapidly rising HCG levels.

▸ Classic ultrasound finding is an echogenic intrauterine lesion with multiple anechoic cystic spaces ("snowstorm" or "cluster of grapes" appearance).

▸ Low-resistance increased vascularity is often identified in a molar pregnancy.

▸ Molar pregnancy is associated with multiple theca luteal cysts due to ovarian hyperstimulation.

▸ Elevated HCG levels 6 months after evacuation of a mole are concerning for invasive or metastatic disease.

▸ Invasive moles extend into the myometrium but do not metastasize.

▸ Choriocarcinomas commonly metastasize to the lungs.

Management

▸ Dilation and evacuation; chemotherapy for invasive or metastatic disease

Further Reading

Green CL, Angtuaco TL, Shah HR, Parmley TH. Gestational trophoblastic disease: a spectrum of radiologic diagnosis. *Radiographics*. 1996;16(6):1371–1384.

History

► 39-year-old woman with pelvic pain and secondary amenorrhea

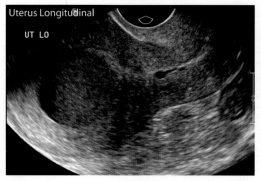

Figure 107.1

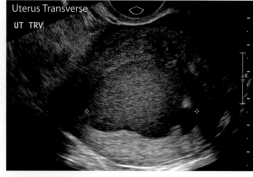

Figure 107.2

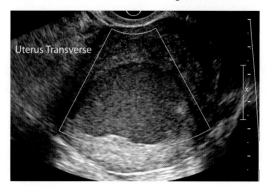

Figure 107.3

Case 107 Hematometra

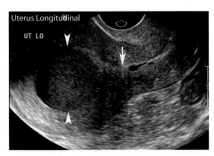

Figure 107.4

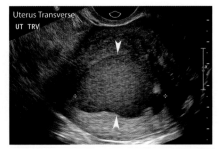

Figure 107.5

Findings

▶ Longitudinal (Figure 107.1) and transverse (Figures 107.2 and 107.3) endovaginal ultrasound images through the uterus show distention of the uterine cavity by an avascular collection with dense internal echoes and increased through transmission (arrowheads in Figures 107.4 and 107.5). Lower uterine segment and visualized endocervical canal are unremarkable (arrow in Figure 107.4).

Differential Diagnosis

▶ Collection within the endometrial cavity may represent blood (hematometra), pus (pyometra), or fluid (hydrometra). The presence of dense internal echoes excludes simple fluid. Hematometra and pyometra both have similar imaging appearance, but pyometra can be excluded here due to lack of clinical signs of infection. Congenital anomalies such as imperforate hymen can cause hematometra, but they usually present in younger females with primary amenorrhea. Acquired hematometra presents with secondary amenorrhea and occurs due to obstruction of the cervix or lower uterine segment by adhesions/scarring after surgery or tumor. No obvious obstructing tumor is seen here. In this adult patient, the hematometra was due to cervical/endometrial adhesions following endometrial ablation.

Teaching Points

▶ Obstruction in the lower genital tract results in accumulation of blood within the endometrial cavity (hematometra or hematocolpometra).
▶ The typical clinical presentation is a female with primary or secondary amenorrhea.
▶ In children/adolescents, congenital anomalies such as imperforate hymen or transverse vaginal septum are the most common causes. Obstruction at the level of the vagina causes hematocolpometra (accumulation of blood in the uterus and vagina).
▶ Scarring and adhesions due to cervical surgery, radiation, endometrial ablation, dilation, or curettage cause secondary hematometra in adults.
▶ Cervical and endometrial malignancies can obstruct the uterine cavity and cause hematometra. Obstructing malignancy needs to be excluded in adults.

Management

▶ Cervical dilation

Further Reading

McCausland AM, McCausland VM. Long-term complications of endometrial ablation: cause, diagnosis, treatment, and prevention. *J Minim Invasive Gynecol.* 2007;14(4):399–406.

History

▶ Radiographs from two patients with history of intrauterine contraceptive device (IUD) placement and pelvic pain

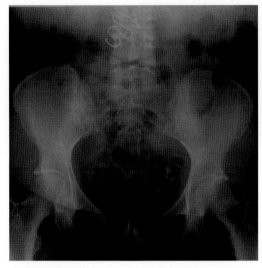

Figure 108.1

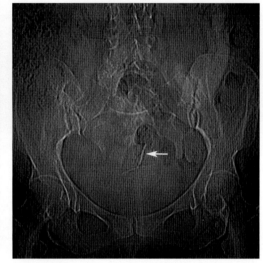

Figure 108.2

Case 108 Misplaced Intrauterine Contraceptive Device

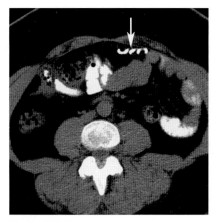

Figure 108.3

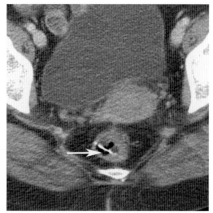

Figure 108.4

Findings

▶ Figure 108.1 shows a curved Lippes loop IUD in the mid-abdomen. Corresponding CT image (Figure 108.3) shows the IUD to be in the anterior peritoneal cavity (arrow).

▶ Figure 108.2 (scout radiograph) shows a T-shaped IUD in the pelvis (arrow). Corresponding CT image (Figure 108.4) shows that the IUD is extrauterine and eroded into the rectum (arrow).

Differential Diagnosis

▶ In the first patient, the location of the IUD in the mid-abdomen is cranial to the expected location of the uterus, which is suspicious for uterine perforation. Subsequent CT confirms the intraperitoneal location consistent with uterine perforation.

▶ In the second patient, it is not possible to assess intra- or extrauterine location on the basis of a single projection scout radiograph. Subsequent CT shows the IUD in the rectum, which is consistent with uterine and subsequent bowel perforation.

Teaching Points

▶ The inability to identify the string of an IUD on physical examination may be due to expulsion of the IUD, detachment of the string, or uterine perforation.

▶ Ultrasound is commonly used to assess the position of the IUD. A normally positioned IUD should have one end within the fundal endometrium and the other proximal to the internal os.

▶ Misplaced IUDs not visualized on ultrasound are assessed by radiograph. CT is not routinely used but can help in accurate localization.

▶ Incidence of uterine perforation of IUD is 1–2 per 1000.

▶ Perforated IUDs may remain in the peritoneal cavity or subsequently perforate into the bowel or bladder.

▶ IUDs positioned low in the uterine cavity may be ineffective and may require repositioning.

▶ Extension of the IUD into the myometrium can cause pelvic pain. It is identified on ultrasound as extension of the echogenic IUD beyond the endometrium into the myometrium.

▶ Presence of the IUD is associated with increased risk of pelvic inflammatory disease.

▶ Pregnancy associated with IUD is often ectopic.

Management

▶ Laparoscopic retrieval

Further Reading
Peri N, Graham D, Levine D. Imaging of intrauterine contraceptive devices. *J Ultrasound Med.* 2007;26(10):1389–1401.

History

► 35-year-old woman with infertility

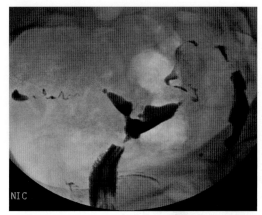

Figure 109.1

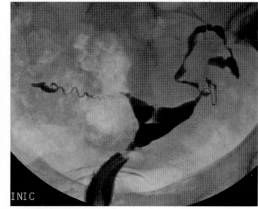

Figure 109.2

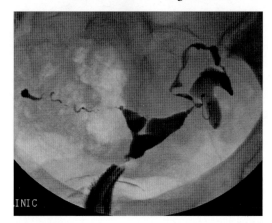

Figure 109.3

Case 109   Uterine Synechiae

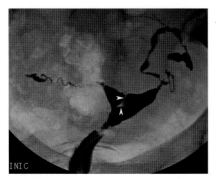

Figure 109.4

Findings

▶ Sequential hysterosalpingogram (HSG) images show opacification of the uterine cavity and bilateral fallopian tubes (Figures 109.1–109.3). Contrast outlines linear filling defects extending from the uterine walls on all three images (arrowheads in Figure 109.4). Loculated intraperitoneal spillage of contrast is noted on the left side.

Differential Diagnosis

▶ Filling defects in the uterine cavity during HSG can be due to endometrial polyps, submucosal fibroids, and intrauterine adhesions (or synechiae). Polyps appear as well-defined round intrauterine filling defects. Submucosal fibroids also cause round filling defects that are often indistinguishable from polyps. Linear filling defects in the uterine cavity, as noted here, are characteristic of uterine synechiae.

Teaching Points

▶ Intrauterine synechiae or adhesions are formed due to scarring and cause infertility.
▶ Interventions such as curettage are the most common cause of uterine synechiae formation.
▶ Endometrial infections can also cause synechiae formation.
▶ Asherman syndrome refers to the clinical syndrome of pain, menstrual disturbance, and/or subfertility in the presence of intrauterine adhesions.
▶ Synechiae appear as linear intrauterine filling defects on HSG.
▶ Hysteroscopy is used to confirm diagnosis and treat the condition.

Management

▶ Hysteroscopic lysis of adhesions

Further Reading

Roma Dalfó A, Ubeda B, Ubeda A, et al. Diagnostic value of hysterosalpingography in the detection of intrauterine abnormalities: a comparison with hysteroscopy. *AJR Am J Roentgenol*. 2004;183(5):1405–1409.

History

▶ 28-year-old woman with infertility

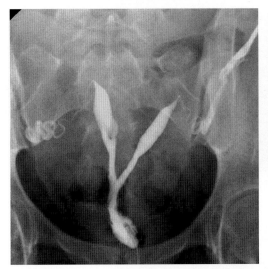

Figure 110.1

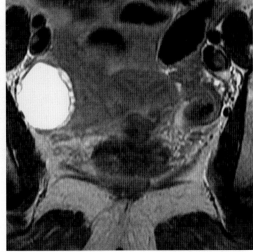

Figure 110.2

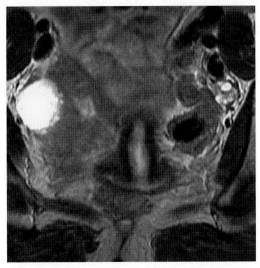

Figure 110.3

Case 110 Septate Uterus

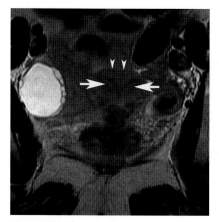

Figure 110.4

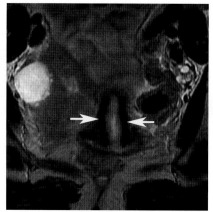

Figure 110.5

Findings

► Hysterosalpingogram (Figure 110.1) reveals two separate symmetric uterine cavities that join caudally at the isthmus with a single cervix. Fallopian tubes are normal appearing, with intraperitoneal spillage seen only on the left at this stage of injection.

► Axial T2-weighted MR image through the uterine body (Figure 110.2) shows two endometrial canals (arrows in Figure 110.4) and a convex uterine fundus (arrowheads in Figure 110.4). An incidental simple right ovarian cyst is present.

► A more caudal axial T2-weighted MR image (Figure 110.3) shows a single cervix (arrows in Figure 110.5).

Differential Diagnosis

► Differential diagnosis of two uterine cavities on imaging includes arcuate, septate, bicornuate uterus, and uterus didelphys. Arcuate morphology can be excluded as it has a single cavity with a depression of the uterine fundal contour on hysterosalpingogram and not the deep acute angle between the uterine cavities noted here. Uterus didelphys has uterine, cervical, and often upper vaginal duplication. Septate and bicornuate morphologies demonstrate two uterine cavities. On hysterosalpingogram, acute intercornual angle (<105) favors septate uterus over bicornuate; however, there is a large degree of overlap and both entities are often indistinguishable. In this patient, normal fundal convexity demonstrated on MR image excludes bicornuate uterus (which has separate horns with a myometrial notch between them) and establishes the diagnosis of septate uterus.

Teaching Points

► Fallopian tubes, uterus, cervix, and the upper two-thirds of the vagina are formed from paired mullerian ducts.
► Incomplete fusion of mullerian ducts results in bicornuate uterus and uterus didelphys.
► Incomplete septal resorption after fusion of mullerian ducts causes septate uterus.
► Septate uterus comprises 55% of congenital uterine anomalies.
► Patients with septate uterus often present with infertility, recurrent abortions, or preterm delivery.
► The septum may be partial or extend up to the external os (complete).
► The septum may be fibrous or muscular.
► Septate uterus is differentiated from bicornuate uterus primarily by normal external fundal contour.

Management

► Surgical excision of septum to treat infertility

Further Reading

Troiano RN, McCarthy SM. Mullerian duct anomalies: imaging and clinical issues. *Radiology.* 2004;233(1):19–34.

History

▶ Hysterosalpingogram (HSG) and pelvic MR images from two women for work-up of mullerian abnormality

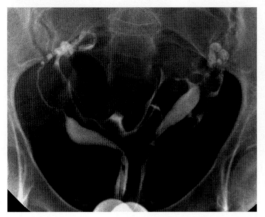

Figure 111.1

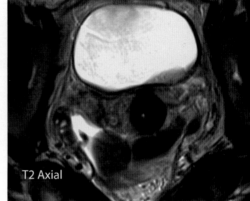

Figure 111.2

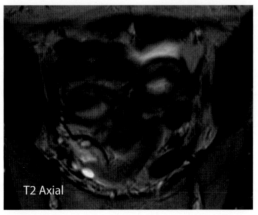

Figure 111.3

Case 111 Uterus Didelphys

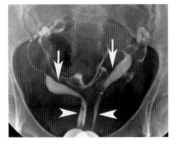
Figure 111.4

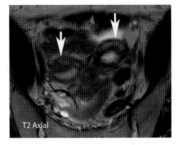
Figure 111.5

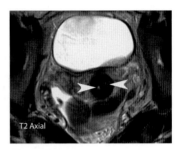
Figure 111.6

Findings

► HSG image (Figure 111.1) shows opacification of two separate cervices and uterine cavities (arrowheads and arrows respectively in Figure 111.4) without any communication of the uterine cavities. Cannulation and simultaneous injection of both cervices was performed to obtain this image.

► Axial T2-weighted MR image (Figure 111.2) shows two separate splayed uterine cavities (arrows in Figure 111.5). A more caudal image (Figure 111.3) shows two fused cervices (arrowheads in Figure 111.6). Zonal anatomy of cervices is identified around the cervical canals.

Differential Diagnosis

► Identification of two divergent uterine horns without any communication and two cervices is diagnostic of uterus didelphys. On MRI, didelphys demonstrates duplication of zonal anatomy of the cervices. Bicornuate uterus has divergent symmetric horns (>105 intercornual angle on HSG) with communication of the uterine cavities at the level of the isthmus. Bicornuate unicollis has a single cervix, while bicornuate bicollis anatomy has duplication of cervix. There is communication between the uterine horns in bicornuate bicollis, differentiating it from didelphys. Septate uterus is identified by normal uterine fundal contour on MR imaging and acute intercornual angle on HSG.

Teaching Points

► Uterus didelphys results due to complete failure of fusion of mullerian ducts.
► It constitutes 5% of uterine anomalies.
► Longitudinal vaginal septum is present in the majority of cases.
► Imaging features include divergent horns, lack of communication between the two uterine cavities, and presence of two cervices with preserved zonal anatomy.
► Spontaneous abortion and premature birth are complications of uterine didelphys.
► Congenital renal abnormalities (most commonly agenesis) are associated with mullerian abnormalities. Unicornuate uterus has the highest incidence of renal abnormalities.

Management

► Metroplasty for patients with spontaneous abortions

Further Reading
Troiano RN, McCarthy SM. Mullerian duct anomalies: imaging and clinical issues. *Radiology.* 2004;233(1):19–34.

History

▶ MRI (Figures 112.1–112.4) and ultrasound (Figures 112.5 and 112.6) images of two patients with pelvic pain

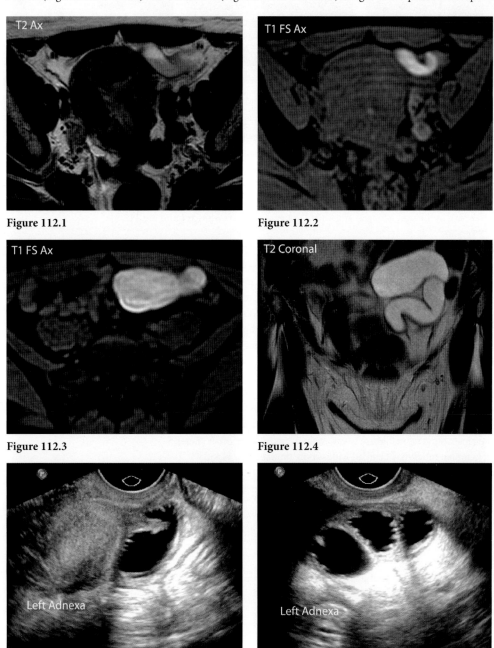

Figure 112.1

Figure 112.2

Figure 112.3

Figure 112.4

Figure 112.5

Figure 112.6

Case 112   Hematosalpinx

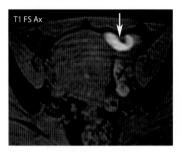

Figure 112.7

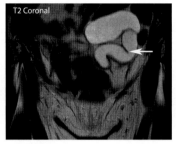

Figure 112.8

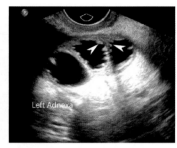

Figure 112.9

Findings

▶ T1- and T2-weighted axial MR images through the pelvis (Figures 112.1 and 112.2) show a T1 and T2 hyperintense dilated tubular structure adjacent to the left uterine cornu (arrow in Figure 112.7). A more cranial image (Figure 112.3) shows a dilated and sac-like component. T2-weighted coronal MR image (Figure 112.4) reveals a tortuous, dilated tubular configuration that is folded on itself (arrow in Figure 112.8).

▶ Transvaginal ultrasound image from a different patient (Figure 112.5) shows a dilated C-shaped cystic structure in the left adnexa. Cross-sectional image through the lesion (Figure 112.6) shows prominent nodular fold thickening in the wall giving a "cogwheel" appearance (arrowheads in Figure 112.9).

Differential Diagnosis

▶ Ovarian cysts constitute the vast majority of adnexal cystic lesions, but dilated fallopian tubes also have a cystic appearance and can be misinterpreted as ovarian cysts. The elongated tubular C- or S-shaped configuration seen here is characteristic of a dilated tube; ovarian cysts have a round configuration. Identification of ipsilateral ovary separate from the dilated tube helps establish the diagnosis of hydrosalpinx. The T1 hyperintensity noted here is consistent with blood products within the dilated tube (hematosalpinx).

▶ Chronic inflammation in a fallopian tube causes thickening of the longitudinal folds. On ultrasound, this gives the beaded or "cogwheel" appearance seen here, which is pathognomic of hydrosalpinx.

Teaching Points

▶ Hydrosalpinx occurs due to obstruction of the distal tube.
▶ Pelvic inflammatory disease is the most common cause of hydrosalpinx.
▶ Endometriosis, surgery, malignancy, and tubal pregnancy are other causes.
▶ Dilated fallopian tubes may be filled with simple fluid, pus, or blood.
▶ Hematosalpinx is usually secondary to endometriosis.
▶ Pyosalpinx or hydrosalpinx can be associated with tubo-ovarian abscess.

Management

▶ Treatment of underlying infection or endometriosis

Further Reading
Kim MY, Rha SE, Oh SN, et al. MR imaging findings of hydrosalpinx: a comprehensive review. *Radiographics*. 2009;29(2):495–507.

Case 113

History

- 45-year-old female with vaginal bleeding

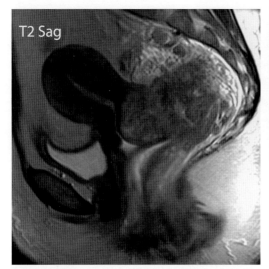

T2 Sag
Figure 113.1

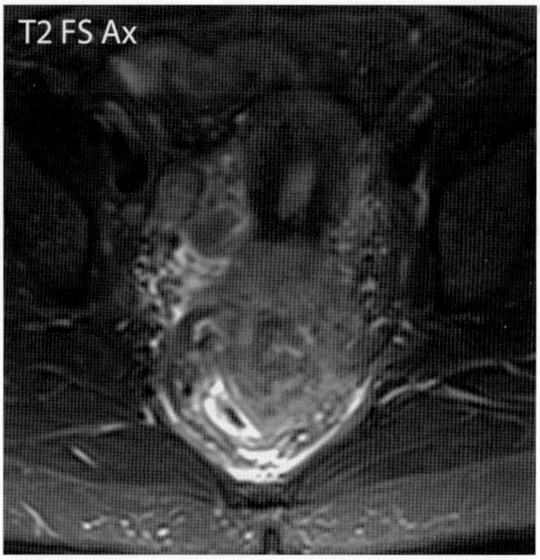

T2 FS Ax
Figure 113.2

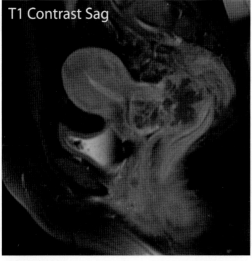

T1 Contrast Sag
Figure 113.3

T1 Ax Contrast
Figure 113.4

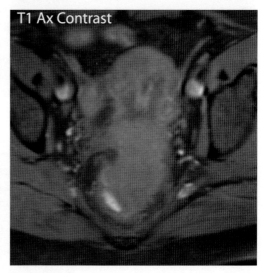

Case 113 Cervical Cancer

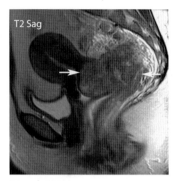
Figure 113.5

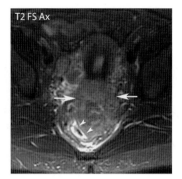
Figure 113.6

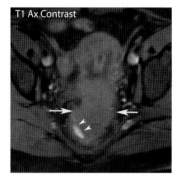
Figure 113.7

Findings

▶ Sagittal T2 (Figure 113.1), fat-suppressed axial T2 (Figure 113.2), and sagittal (Figure 113.3) and axial (Figure 113.4) contrast-enhanced MR images of the pelvis are shown. A large exophytic T2 hyperintense, heterogeneously enhancing mass arises from the posterior lip of the cervix (arrows in Figure 113.5). The mass extends beyond the cervix into the parametrium (arrows in Figures 113.6 and 113.7). Rectal involvement is present with loss of intervening fat plane (arrowheads).

Differential Diagnosis

▶ MR imaging is used for staging cervical cancer and accurately assesses tumor size, depth of invasion, and pelvic lymphadenopathy. Stage I disease is confined to the cervix. Stage II disease has upper vaginal involvement. Stage IIA does not have parametrial invasion, while stage IIB has parametrial extension. Stage IIIA disease has lower vaginal involvement, while stage IIIB has extension to the pelvic sidewall or hydronephrosis. Extension to the bladder or rectum is stage IVA, while distant metastasis is IVB.

▶ In this patient, the T2 hyperintense mass obliterates the T2 hypointense cervical stroma, extends into the parametrium, and invades the rectum. The rectal involvement makes this stage IVA cervical cancer.

Teaching Points

▶ Risk factors for cervical cancer include human papillomavirus infection and multiple sexual partners.

▶ Squamous cell carcinoma comprises 80%–90% and adenocarcinoma 10%–20% of cervical malignancies.

▶ Cervical cancer presents with vaginal bleeding and most frequently occurs in women aged 45–55 years.

▶ MR imaging accurately differentiates early cervical cancer (stage I/IIA), which is treated surgically; more advanced disease requires radiation/chemotherapy.

▶ Cervical cancer is T2 hyperintense, which helps differentiate it from T2 hypointense cervical stroma. A break in the T2 hypointense ring of cervical stroma by the tumor suggests extension into the parametrium.

▶ PET-CT can help in staging and detecting residual/recurrent disease.

▶ Ultrasound is not useful for detecting or staging cervical cancer.

Management

▶ Surgery (early disease) and radiation/chemotherapy (advanced disease)

Further Reading
Sala E, Wakely S, Senior E, Lomas D. MRI of malignant neoplasms of the uterine corpus and cervix. *AJR Am J Roentgenol.* 2007;188(6):1577–1587.

Case 114

History

- Pelvic ultrasound (Figure 114.1) and MR images (Figures 114.2–114.4) from two patients with postmenopausal bleeding

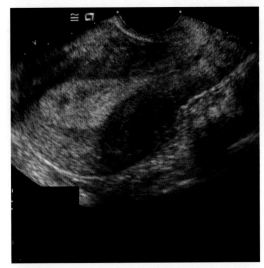

Figure 114.1

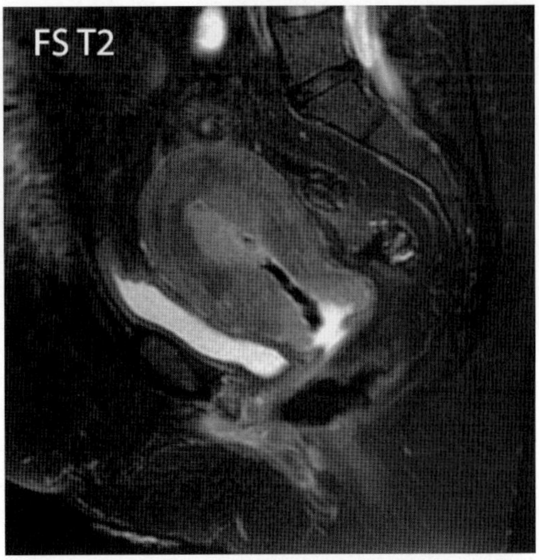

FS T2

Figure 114.2

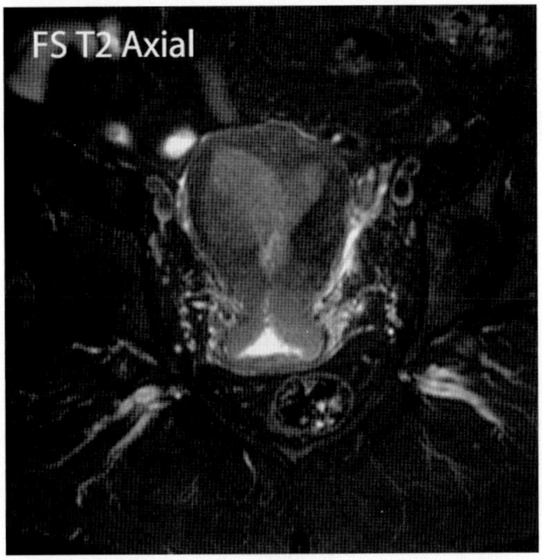

FS T2 Axial

Figure 114.3

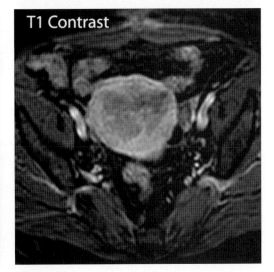

T1 Contrast

Figure 114.4

Case 114 Endometrial Cancer

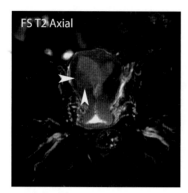
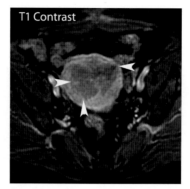

Figure 114.5   **Figure 114.6**

Findings

▶ Longitudinal ultrasound image (Figure 114.1) reveals a thickened heterogeneous endometrium.

▶ Sagittal and axial T2-weighted images (Figures 114.2 and 114.3) show expansion of the endometrium by isointense endometrial tumor. Tumor extension into myometrium is noted (arrowheads in Figure 114.5). Myometrial invasion by hypoenhancing tumor is identified after contrast administration (Figure 114.4, arrowheads in Figure 114.6).

Differential Diagnosis

▶ Differential diagnosis of endometrial thickening (>5 mm) on ultrasound in postmenopausal bleeding includes endometrial hyperplasia, polyp, cancer, and tamoxifen-associated changes. Endometrial thickening due to cancer is irregular and heterogeneous, but these features are nonspecific. Endometrial biopsy confirms the diagnosis.

▶ MR imaging stages endometrial cancer by identifying the depth of myometrial invasion. In this patient, the tumor has invaded >50% of the myometrium, which is consistent with stage IB disease. Endometrial hyperplasia and cancer cannot be differentiated on MR imaging.

Teaching Points

▶ Postmenopausal bleeding with endometrial thickening >5 mm or any focal thickening on ultrasound should be evaluated with biopsy, hysteroscopy, or sonohysterography to assess for cancer.

▶ Ninety percent of endometrial malignancies are adenocarcinomas.

▶ The majority (about 75%) occur in postmenopausal women. Abnormal vaginal bleeding is the predominant presentation.

▶ The 2009 FIGO staging for endometrial cancer defines tumor confined to the uterus with <50% myometrial invasion as stage IA and with >50% invasion as stage IB. Cervical stromal involvement is stage II. Stage III has serosal/adnexal involvement (IIIA), vaginal/parametrial involvement (IIIB), or pelvic/para-aortic lymph node involvement (IIIC). Bladder/bowel involvement or distant metastasis is stage IV.

▶ On T2 imaging, endometrial cancer is hyperintense to myometrium and iso- to hypointense to endometrium. It is hypoenhancing to myometrium after contrast administration.

▶ The depth of myometrial involvement (stage IA/IB) is an important prognostic factor and is well assessed by MR imaging. Cervical stromal and adjacent organ involvement can also be assessed.

▶ Irregularity of the endometrial–myometrial junction suggests invasion.

Management

▶ Surgery with or without adjuvant therapy

Further Reading

Beddy P, O'Neill AC, Yamamoto AK, Addley HC, Reinhold C, Sala E. FIGO staging system for endometrial cancer: added benefits of MR imaging. *Radiographics*. 2012;32(1):241–254.

History

▶ 25-year-old female with abdominal pain and positive pregnancy test

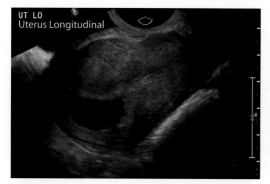

Figure 115.1

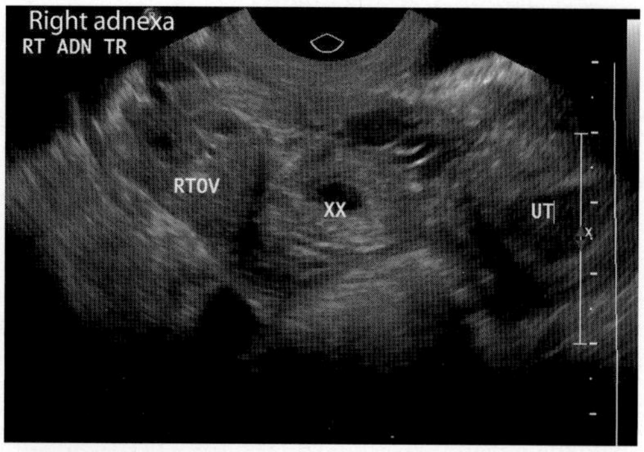

Figure 115.2

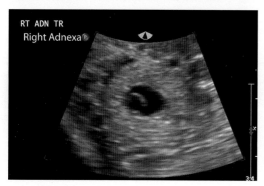

Figure 115.3

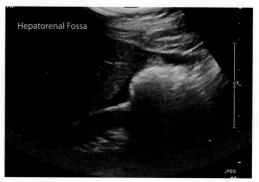

Figure 115.4

Case 115 Ectopic Pregnancy

Findings

▶ Longitudinal ultrasound image of the uterus (Figure 115.1) shows an irregular intrauterine fluid collection lined by a thin echogenic rim.

▶ Transverse ultrasound image of right adnexa (Figure 115.2) shows an echogenic structure with central anechoic component (marked XX) located between the right ovary (RTOV) and uterus (UT).

▶ Figure 115.3 is a magnified image of the left adnexal lesion. The central anechoic component has a small yolk sac with possible embryo.

▶ The image of the hepatorenal fossa demonstrates free abdominal fluid (Figure 115.4).

Differential Diagnosis

▶ In this patient with positive pregnancy test, the intrauterine fluid collection without yolk sac or fetal pole may represent very early intrauterine pregnancy, blighted ovum, or pseudogestational sac of ectopic pregnancy. The irregular shape of collection, large size without identifiable yolk sac, and thin rim make viable intrauterine pregnancy extremely unlikely. The presence of an adnexal lesion separate from the ovary is consistent with an ectopic, with the endometrial collection representing a pseudogestational sac. Intraperitoneal free fluid raises concern of bleeding due to a ruptured ectopic.

Teaching Points

▶ Women with tubal disease, intrauterine contraceptive device, and undergoing infertility treatment are at higher risk for ectopic pregnancy.

▶ Normal intrauterine gestational sacs are regular, round, or oval and have a thick hyperechoic rim (at least 2 mm).

▶ Ectopic pregnancies have associated intrauterine pseudogestational sacs in 10%–20% of patients.

▶ Fallopian tubes are the most common location of ectopic pregnancy.

▶ An adnexal mass separate from the ovary is highly likely to be an ectopic, while a mass within the ovary is likely a corpus luteal cyst.

▶ An effort should be made to apply pressure and move an adnexal mass during ultrasound in order to determine if it moves separate from the ovary.

▶ Fifteen to thirty-five percent of ectopic pregnancies do not have demonstrable adnexal mass on ultrasound. Follow-up is required in all pregnant patients who do not have demonstrable intra- or extrauterine pregnancy.

▶ New guidelines for the evaluation of first trimester pregnancy have been published by Doubilet et al (2013).

Management

▶ Surgery or methotrexate

Further Reading

Doubilet PM, Benson CB, Bourne, et al. Diagnostic criteria for nonviable pregnancy early in the first trimester. *N Engl J Med.* 2013;369(15):1443–1451.

History

▶ 32-year-old female with chronic pelvic pain

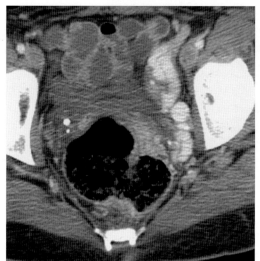

Figure 116.1

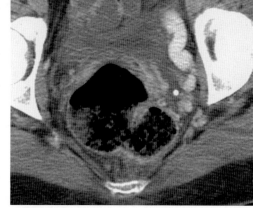

Figure 116.2

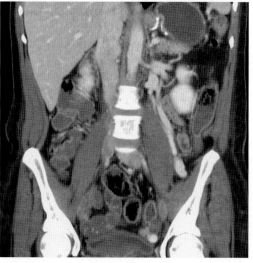

Figure 116.3

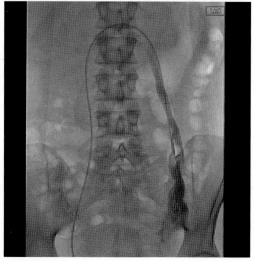

Figure 116.4

Case 116 Pelvic Congestion Syndrome

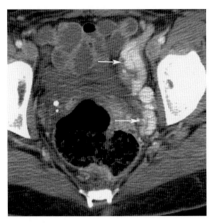
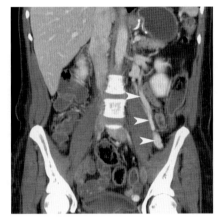

Figure 116.5   **Figure 116.6**

Findings

▶ Contrast-enhanced CT images (Figures 116.1–116.3) show dilated veins along the left pelvic sidewall (arrows in Figure 116.5). A dilated tortuous left ovarian vein is also noted (arrowheads in Figure 116.6)

▶ A venogram (Figure 116.4) shows dilated tortuous left pelvic venous plexus draining into a dilated ovarian vein.

Differential Diagnosis

▶ Differential diagnosis of dilated pelvic veins includes arteriovenous malformation, venous obstruction, pelvic congestion syndrome, and normal asymptomatic variant. Arteriovenous malformations can be identified by early venous opacification during the arterial phase and by the presence of a prominent feeding artery. Asymptomatic dilated pelvic collaterals may be present if there is a history of inferior vena cava or other venous obstruction. Dilated pelvic veins can also be a normal variant in asymptomatic patients. However, in this patient with chronic pelvic pain, the presence of dilated pelvic varices suggests the diagnosis of pelvic congestion syndrome.

Teaching Points

▶ Pelvic congestion syndrome is one of the causes of chronic pelvic pain. It is diagnosed by the presence of ovarian varicosities on imaging in patients with chronic pelvic pain of duration longer than 6 months.

▶ Endometriosis, adenomyosis, and pelvic inflammatory disease are other causes of pelvic pain that need to be excluded before pelvic congestion syndrome is considered.

▶ Dilated pelvic veins can be present in asymptomatic women, and the diagnosis of pelvic congestion syndrome should not be made in the absence of clinical symptoms.

▶ The etiology of pelvic congestion syndrome is unclear but may be secondary to venous valvular incompetence in the iliac and ovarian veins.

▶ Multiparity is a risk factor.

▶ Uterine tenderness, adnexal tenderness, and vulvar varicosities may be present.

▶ Dilated pelvic veins may be demonstrated on CT, MRI, or ultrasound.

Management

▶ If symptomatic, treatment of dilated pelvic collaterals can be performed with transcatheter embolization or surgery.

Further Reading
Rane N, Leyon JJ, Littlehales T, Ganeshan A, Crowe P, Uberoi R. Pelvic congestion syndrome. *Curr Probl Diagn Radiol.* 2013;42(4):135–140.

History

▶ 54-year-old woman on tamoxifen for breast cancer

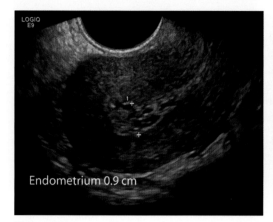

Figure 117.1

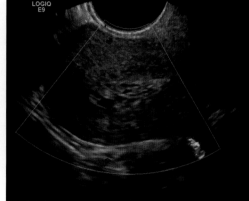

Figure 117.2

Case 117 Tamoxifen-Related Endometrial Changes

Findings

▶ Grayscale and color Doppler images show a thickened endometrium with numerous small cystic spaces in the endometrium (Figures 117.1 and 117.2).

Differential Diagnosis

▶ Thickened endometrium with multiple cystic spaces is a common sonographic pattern seen in postmenopausal women who are receiving tamoxifen; it is most often caused by benign cystic endometrial atrophy. However, this ultrasound appearance is nonspecific, and an array of other tamoxifen-associated conditions including endometrial hyperplasia, endometrial cancer, and endometrial polyp can have a similar ultrasound appearance.

Teaching Points

▶ Tamoxifen has an anti-estrogenic effect in the breast but an estrogenic effect in other tissues including the uterus.
▶ Normal postmenopausal endometrium measures up to 5 mm, but postmenopausal women on tamoxifen therapy often have thickened and cystic endometrium without any serious underlying pathology.
▶ Endometrial cystic atrophy and endometrial polyps are the most common causes of tamoxifen-related endometrial thickening.
▶ Sonohysterography can be used to identify polyps in patients with thickened endometrium.
▶ Tamoxifen increases the risk of endometrial cancer two-fold, and the risk increases with duration of treatment.
▶ Endometrial cancer usually presents with bleeding, and such patients should undergo endometrial biopsy.

Management

▶ Endometrial cystic atrophy is a benign condition, but endometrial cancer needs to be excluded, especially in patients with vaginal bleeding.

Further Reading
Polin SA, Ascher SM. The effect of tamoxifen on the genital tract. *Cancer Imaging*. 2008 30;8:135–145.

History

▶ 29-year-old female with infertility

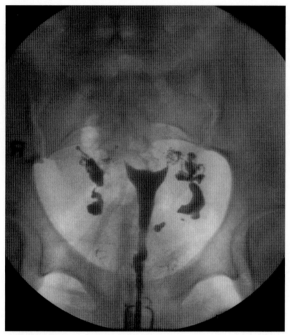

Figure 118.1

Case 118 Salpingitis Isthmica Nodosa

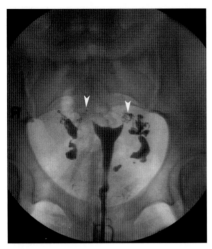

Figure 118.2

Findings

▶ Hysterosalpingogram demonstrates multiple small outpouchings of contrast alongside the bilateral fallopian tubes. The tubes are not well seen in the involved segment (Figures 118.1 and 118.2).

Differential Diagnosis

▶ The presence of multiple tiny outpouchings from the fallopian tubes is diagnostic of salpingitis isthmica nodosa.

Teaching Points

▶ Salpingitis isthmica nodosa is caused by nodular scarring of the fallopian tubes of uncertain etiology, but thought likely due to inflammation.
▶ It commonly affects the isthmic portion of the fallopian tubes, as the name suggests.
▶ It is associated with infertility (37.5%) and ectopic tubal pregnancy (9.4%).
▶ History of pelvic inflammatory disease is a risk factor.

Management

▶ Recanalization or resection of the involved segment may be performed, but this diagnosis has been associated with increased failure rate. However, no consensus on therapy is available.

Further Reading
Creasy JL, Clark RL, Cuttino JT, Groff TR. Salpingitis isthmica nodosa: radiologic and clinical correlates. *Radiology.* 1985;154(3):597–600.

Section IX Ovary

History

▶ 33-year-old woman with pelvic pain

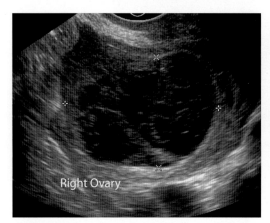

Figure 119.1

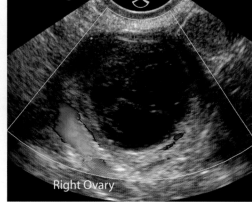

Figure 119.2

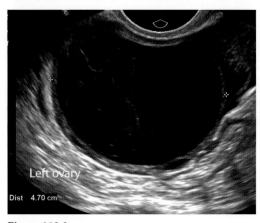

Figure 119.3

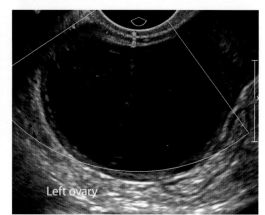

Figure 119.4

Case 119 Hemorrhagic Ovarian Cyst

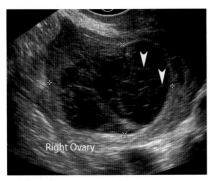

Figure 119.5

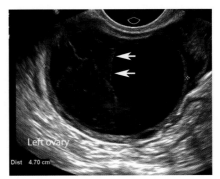

Figure 119.6

Findings

▶ Grayscale and Doppler images of the right ovary (Figures 119.1 and 119.2) show a cystic lesion with a network of thin reticulations (arrowheads in Figure 119.5) giving a "fishnet" appearance. No vascularity is present in the reticulations.

▶ Grayscale and Doppler images of the left ovary (Figures 119.3 and 119.4) show a cystic lesion with a clear anechoic component and an echogenic component. The echogenic component has concave angular margins (arrows in Figure 119.6). Circumferential flow is present in the wall, but no flow is identified within the echogenic component.

Differential Diagnosis

▶ The diagnostic dilemma here is differentiating malignant ovarian cysts from common complex hemorrhagic cysts. Malignant ovarian neoplasms usually occur in postmenopausal women and have thick septations and nodularity, often showing internal vascularity. The fine internal reticulations (right adnexal lesion) and echogenic component with concave angular margins representing a retracting clot (left ovarian lesion) are characteristic features of hemorrhagic cysts in premenopausal women. Absence of internal vascularity also supports this diagnosis.

Teaching Points

▶ Hemorrhagic ovarian cysts develop after ovulation due to rupture of fragile blood vessels in the vascularized granulosa layer.

▶ They occur in premenopausal women and may cause pelvic pain.

▶ Blood in hemorrhagic cysts typically evolves from acute hemorrhage to clot formation to clot retraction, giving characteristic sonographic appearance.

▶ Fine reticular, or fishnet, appearance is the most common sonographic finding and is caused by fibrin strands within the cyst.

▶ Retracting clots are the second most common feature of hemorrhagic cysts and are identified by their concave angular margins and lack of internal vascularity.

▶ Hemorrhagic cysts can have a thick vascular wall.

▶ They usually resolve in 8 weeks.

▶ Typical hemorrhagic cysts (fine internal reticulations or retracting clot) measuring up to 5 cm in premenopausal women do not require follow-up. Larger lesions can be followed in 6–12 weeks (ideally with ultrasound done during the follicular phase).

Management

▶ No follow-up is needed for hemorrhagic cysts up to 5 cm.

Further Reading

Jain KA. Sonographic spectrum of hemorrhagic ovarian cysts. *J Ultrasound Med.* 2002;21(8):879–886.

History

▶ 37-year-old woman with dysmenorrhea

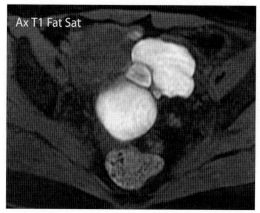

Figure 120.1

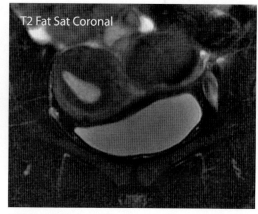

Figure 120.2

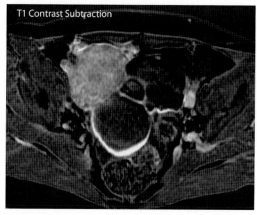

Figure 120.3

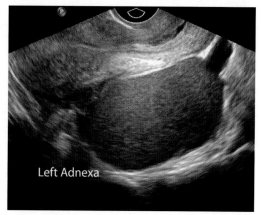

Figure 120.4

Case 120   Ovarian Endometrioma

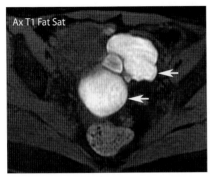

Figure 120.5

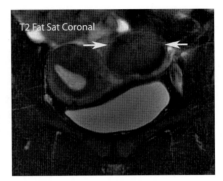

Figure 120.6

Findings

▶ Unenhanced fat-suppressed T1-weighted image of the pelvis (Figure 120.1) shows a multiseptated T1 hyperintense left pelvic lesion (arrows in Figure 120.5).

▶ On coronal fat-suppressed T2-weighted image (Figure 120.2), the left adnexal lesion is hypointense (arrows in Figure 120.6).

▶ Post-contrast subtracted T1-weighted image (Figure 120.3) shows wall but no internal enhancement.

▶ Ultrasound (Figure 120.4) reveals homogeneous internal echoes within the adnexal lesion.

Differential Diagnosis

▶ Differential diagnosis of an adnexal lesion in the reproductive age group includes hemorrhagic cyst, endometrioma, dermoids, and benign and malignant ovarian tumors. High signal on fat-suppressed T1-weighted imaging suggests the presence of blood products, a finding that is present in hemorrhagic cysts and endometriomas. T2 hypointensity noted here is caused by chronic recurrent hemorrhage and is characteristic of endometrioma. Acute/subacute blood in hemorrhagic cysts is not T2 hypointense. Homogeneous internal echoes on ultrasound are also consistent with endometrioma. Hemorrhagic cysts have reticular appearance or demonstrate retracting clots. Multilocularity and thin wall enhancement, which are also seen in neoplasms, can be present in endometriomas and do not exclude the diagnosis. Dermoids are T1 hyperintense on nonfat-suppressed images but hypointense on fat-suppressed sequences.

Teaching Points

▶ Endometriosis is caused by the presence of endometrial glands outside the uterus.

▶ Eighty percent of endometriosis occurs in the ovaries.

▶ Recurrent bleeding into endometriomas causes a high concentration of heme products, giving characteristic high T1 and low T2 signal (91%–98% specific).

▶ Low T2 signal of an endometrioma with high T1 signal is called T2 shading.

▶ High signal on fat-suppressed T1 and T2 imaging is a feature of hemorrhagic cysts but may be seen in endometriomas.

▶ On ultrasound, diffuse low-level internal echoes are present in 95% of endometriomas (specificity 81%).

▶ The presence of punctate echogenic wall foci in addition to low-level internal echoes is very specific (99%) for endometrioma.

Management

▶ Treatment of endometriosis varies with the location and symptoms.

Further Reading
Jeong YY, Outwater EK, Kang HK. Imaging evaluation of ovarian masses. *Radiographics*. 2000;20(5):1445–1470.

History

▶ Incidental pelvic lesions in four women of reproductive age

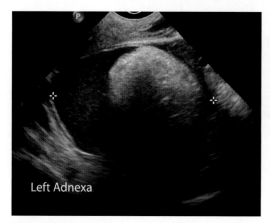

Figure 121.1

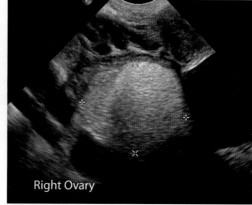

Figure 121.2

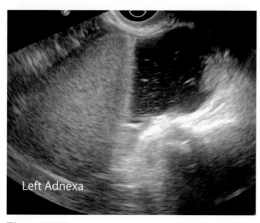

Figure 121.3

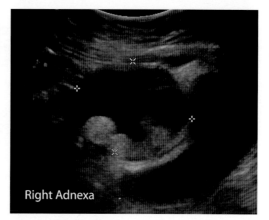

Figure 121.4

Case 121   Ovarian Dermoid Cyst: Mature Cystic Teratoma

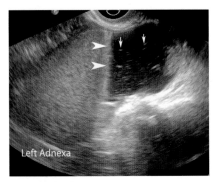

Figure 121.5

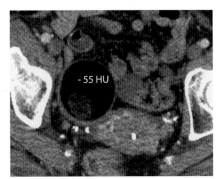

Figure 121.6

Findings

▶ Figure 121.1 shows left adnexal cyst (calipers) containing a highly echogenic focus with dense posterior acoustic shadowing.

▶ Figure 121.2 shows a homogeneous diffusely echogenic adnexal mass (calipers) with posterior acoustic attenuation.

▶ Figure 121.3 reveals a large complex ovarian mass with a fluid level (arrowheads in Figure 121.5). Numerous small hyperechoic lines are present (arrows in Figure 121.5).

▶ Figure 121.4 shows echogenic spherical balls in a cystic cavity.

▶ CT image (Figure 121.6) shows a fat-containing right adnexal lesion.

Differential Diagnosis

▶ The four images depict characteristic ultrasound features of dermoid cysts. Echogenic focus with dense shadowing seen in Figure 121.1 is a characteristic appearance of a Rokitansky protuberance. Diffuse homogeneous increased echogenicity with acoustic shadowing, as seen in Figure 121.2, is due to sebaceous content. Hair in a dermoid causes a typical "hyperechoic-lines-and-dots" appearance, as seen in Figure 121.3. Figure 121.3 also shows a fluid level due to layering of sebum. Figure 121.5 shows spherical echogenic balls that represent a rare but pathognomic appearance of a dermoid cyst. Usually more than one of these patterns is present, allowing for confident identification of most dermoid cysts.

▶ Demonstration of fat in an adnexal tumor by CT or MR imaging is diagnostic of a dermoid cyst.

Teaching Points

▶ Dermoid cysts are common, benign, ovarian, germ cell tumors that contain mature tissues derived from the ectoderm (skin, hair, teeth), mesoderm (fat, bone, muscle), and endoderm (epithelium).

▶ They occur in the younger age group (mean age 30 years) compared with epithelial tumors.

▶ Ten percent are bilateral.

▶ On gross examination, dermoids are unilocular cysts filled with sebaceous material. A protuberance projecting into the cyst cavity (Rokitansky protuberance or dermoid plug) often contains hair, teeth, or bone.

▶ Most patients are asymptomatic.

▶ Torsion, rupture, and rarely malignant transformation can complicate dermoid cysts.

Management

▶ Large symptomatic or complicated dermoids are excised. Smaller asymptomatic tumors are managed conservatively.

Further Reading

Outwater EK, Siegelman ES, Hunt JL. Ovarian teratomas: tumor types and imaging characteristics. *Radiographics.* 2001;21(2):475–490.

History

▶ 53-year-old woman with left pelvic mass

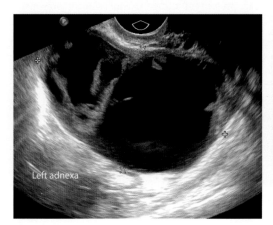

Figure 122.1

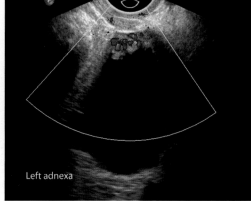

Figure 122.2

Case 122 Ovarian Cancer

Findings

▶ Grayscale and color Doppler images (Figures 122.1 and 122.2) of the pelvis show a large multilocular cystic left adnexal mass with thick irregular septa, multiple papillary projections, and peripheral solid components. Vascularity is noted within the papillary projections.

Differential Diagnosis

▶ Absence of typical findings excludes common benign diagnoses such as hemorrhagic cyst (reticular pattern, retracting clot), endometrioma (low-level internal echoes), hydrosalpinx (tubular shape, cogwheel appearance), and dermoid (hyperechoic mass, acoustic shadowing, hyperechoic lines and dots). Ovarian neoplastic cysts can be benign (cystadenoma) or malignant (carcinoma). While simple cysts are always benign, the probability of malignancy progressively increases with increasing septations, multilocularity, papillary projections, and solid components. In this patient, the presence of thick irregular septa, papillary projections larger than 3 mm, and solid components is very worrisome for ovarian carcinoma. Peripheral vascularity can be present in benign cystic lesions, but vascularity in the solid component or papillary excrescence (as noted here) is a feature of malignancy.

Teaching Points

▶ Ovarian tumors can be epithelial, germ cell, sex cord, stromal, or metastatic in origin.
▶ Epithelial tumors (mainly serous and mucinous carcinomas) account for 85%–90% of ovarian malignancies.
▶ Epithelial ovarian malignancies occur mainly in those in the postmenopausal age group.
▶ Presentation is often late with metastatic disease.
▶ Ovarian carcinomas metastasize by peritoneal seeding (most common) or lymphatic spread. Hematogenous spread occurs only in advanced disease.
▶ Morphologic features on ultrasound can predict malignancy with sensitivity of 85%–97% and specificity of 58%–95%.
▶ Overlap exists between the Doppler waveform of benign inflammatory disease and malignancy. The main role of Doppler imaging is to identify vascularity in solid components/septations that would favor malignancy.
▶ CT plays a limited role in evaluating adnexal lesions but is used to assess the extent of metastatic disease.
▶ Adnexal MRI is mainly used to identify endometriomas, dermoids, and leiomyomas that have atypical ultrasound appearance. The superior soft tissue resolution of MRI demonstrates enhancing septations, nodularity, and solid components present in ovarian malignancies.

Management

▶ Surgery for resection and staging

Further Reading

Twickler DM, Moschos E. Ultrasound and assessment of ovarian cancer risk. *AJR Am J Roentgenol.* 2010;194(2):322–329.

History

▶ 37-year-old woman with palpable left pelvic lump

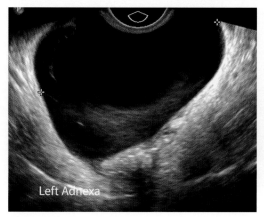

Figure 123.1

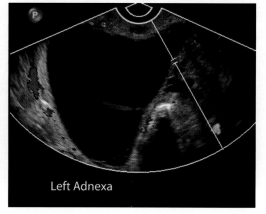

Figure 123.2

Case 123   Ovarian Cystadenoma

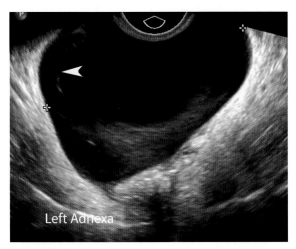

Figure 123.3

Findings

▶ Grayscale and color Doppler images of the left adnexa (Figures 123.1 and 123.2) show a large smooth-walled unilocular ovarian cyst. A thin internal septation is noted (arrow in Figure 123.3). Vascularity is identified along the cyst wall but not within the internal septation.

Differential Diagnosis

▶ Simple ovarian cysts are benign; progressively increasing complexity increases the probability of malignancy. Absence of features of malignancy (thick septations >3 mm, solid elements with flow, focal wall thickening >3 mm) makes ovarian cancer less likely in this patient. The presence of few thin (<3 mm) septations is considered an indeterminate feature in an ovarian cyst and suggests a benign neoplastic process, most commonly a serous or mucinous cystadenoma. It is not possible to differentiate between these two entities on ultrasound; however, serous cystadenoma may be uni- or multilocular, while mucinous cystadenoma is typically multilocular.

Teaching Points

▶ Ovarian epithelial tumors are classified as benign (60%), malignant (35%), or borderline (5%).
▶ Benign serous cystadenomas are the most common ovarian epithelial neoplasm and comprise 60% of ovarian serous tumors.
▶ Benign mucinous cystadenomas constitute 80% of all mucinous ovarian neoplasms.
▶ Cystadenomas occur commonly in the fourth and fifth decades.
▶ Serous cystadenomas are usually unilocular and comprise 84% of simple cysts, which are surgically removed.
▶ Cystadenomas usually have smooth walls and may contain thin septations. Papillary projections, a characteristic of ovarian malignancy, are absent.

Management

▶ Cysts with indeterminate features such as thin septations are surgically removed if they do not resolve after a short-term follow-up study.

Further Reading

Jung SE, Lee JM, Rha SE, Byun JY, Jung JI, Hahn ST. CT and MR imaging of ovarian tumors with emphasis on differential diagnosis. *Radiographics*. 2002;22(6):1305–1325

History

▶ 35-year-old female with gastric mass

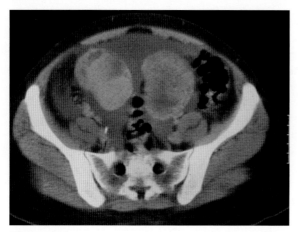

Figure 124.1

Case 124 Bilateral Ovarian Metastases

Findings

▶ Contrast-enhanced CT image (Figure 124.1) shows heterogeneously enhancing adnexal masses with a moderate amount of pelvis free fluid.

Differential Diagnosis

▶ Bilateral enhancing ovarian masses can represent primary ovarian malignancy or metastases from a separate primary such as breast or gastrointestinal tract. Although there is overlap in the imaging appearance, metastases to ovary are often bilateral, solid, and enhancing, while primary ovarian malignancies are usually cystic. In this patient with known primary gastric cancer, the bilateral involvement and solid enhancing nature of the adnexal lesions are highly suggestive of ovarian metastases. Ovarian endometriomas are bilateral in 19%–28% of patients, but do not have the solid enhancing components seen here.

Teaching Points

▶ Breast, stomach, and colon are common primaries that can metastasize to the ovaries.
▶ Spread to the ovaries can be hematogeneous (breast primary) or peritoneal (stomach or other gastrointestinal primary).
▶ Kruckenberg tumor refers to ovarian signet cell metastases from gastric cancer, although it is commonly used as a descriptor for other types of ovarian metastases.
▶ Breast and stomach primaries have solid/predominantly solid ovarian metastasis, while colon primaries are more often cystic.

Management

▶ Excision and/or chemotherapy

Further Reading
Gore RM, Newmark GM, Thakrar KH, Mehta UK, Berlin JW. Pelvic incidentalomas. *Cancer Imaging*. 2010 Oct 4;10 Spec no A:S15–2S6.

History

▶ 45-year-old female with incidental left pelvic mass

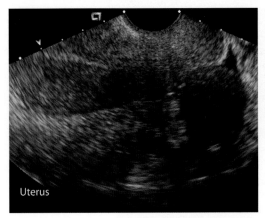

Figure 125.1

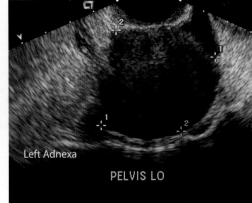

Figure 125.2

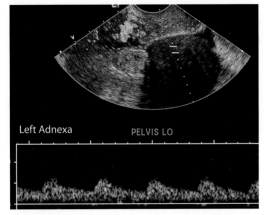

Figure 125.3

125 Ovarian Fibroma

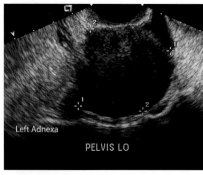

Figure 125.4

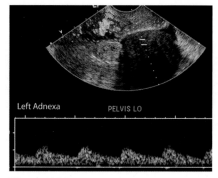

Figure 125.5

Findings

▶ Grayscale and color Doppler images of the pelvis (Figures 125.1–125.5) show a homogeneous hypoechoic left adnexal lesion with posterior acoustic shadowing and internal vascularity.

Differential Diagnosis

▶ Posterior acoustic shadowing and internal vascularity confirm the solid nature of this homogeneous hypoechoic adnexal mass. Solid adnexal masses are unusual, and the differential includes primary tumors such as ovarian fibroma, Brenner tumor, and dysgerminoma; metastasis; and exophytic uterine fibroid. It may be difficult to distinguish a pedunculated exophytic fibroid from a solid ovarian neoplasm. The presence of additional similar-appearing fibroids, demonstration of a vascular pedicle from the uterus that leads to the mass, and, most important, separate identification of the ovaries help in the diagnosis of exophytic fibroids. Ovarian metastases are often bilateral with a known primary tumor. Ovarian fibromas present as solid homogeneous hypoechoic masses on ultrasound. However, Brenner tumors and dysgerminomas may have a similar imaging appearance. An ovarian fibroma was confirmed on histopathology in this patient.

Teaching Points

▶ Ovarian fibroma, fibrothecoma, and thecoma are a spectrum of benign sex cord stromal tumors.
▶ Fibromas are composed of fibroblasts, while estrogen-producing lipid-rich thecomas have fewer fibroblasts.
▶ Fibromas are often asymptomatic unilateral tumors in pre- and postmenopausal women.
▶ Fibromas are associated with ascites and pleural effusions (Meig's syndrome).
▶ On ultrasound, they are homogeneous hypoechoic solid masses with post-acoustic shadowing.
▶ Due to their fibrous component, they are low signal on T1- and T2-weighted MRI. Low signal on T2-weighted MRI of an ovarian tumor is suggestive of a fibroma, although fibroids also have low T2 signal.
▶ Fibromas have delayed mild enhancement after contrast administration. This may help differentiate from fibroids that enhance similar to the myometrium.

Management

▶ Fibromas are benign tumors. However, they are usually surgically resected, as confident preoperative differentiation from malignant entities may not be possible.

Further Reading

Jung SE, Lee JM, Rha SE, Byun JY, Jung JI, Hahn ST. CT and MR imaging of ovarian tumors with emphasis on differential diagnosis. *Radiographics*. 2002;*22*(6):1305–1325.

Case 126

History

► 36-year-old female with right pelvic pain

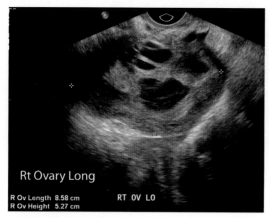

Figure 126.1

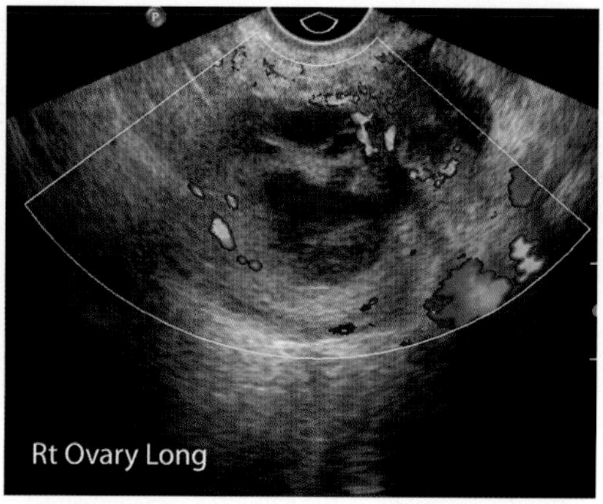

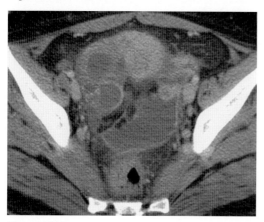

Figure 126.2

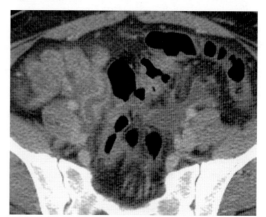

Figure 126.3

Figure 126.4

Case 126 Tubo-ovarian Abscess

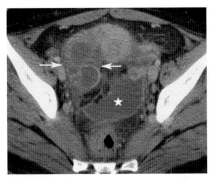

Figure 126.5

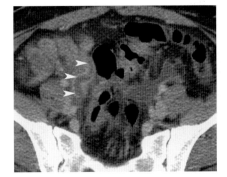

Figure 126.6

Findings

▶ Grayscale and color Doppler ultrasound images (Figures 126.1 and 126.2) reveal a large 8.6 × 5.3 cm thick-walled right adnexal complex lesion with cystic spaces, debris, and vascularity. The right ovary was not visualized separately. The left ovary was normal (not shown),

▶ Contrast CT (Figure 126.3) shows a complex right adnexal lesion (arrows in Figure 126.5) with indistinct margins, cystic areas, and pelvic fat stranding. Rim-enhancing partially loculated pelvic fluid collection (asterisk) is present.

▶ Figure 126.4 shows a right adnexal tubular fluid-filled structure (arrowheads in Figure 126.6).

Differential Diagnosis

▶ Differential diagnosis of complex adnexal lesion includes ovarian neoplasm, hemorrhagic cyst, endometrioma, and tubo-ovarian abscess (TOA). Hemorrhagic cysts (fishnet reticulations, retracting clots) and endometriomas (low-level internal echoes) are identified by their ultrasound characteristics and can be excluded. TOA and ovarian neoplasms can both present as complex multicystic adnexal lesions. Thick walls, debris, and increased vascularity are features of TOA, but it is the identification of a tubular right adnexal structure on CT representing a dilated fallopian tube that clinches the diagnosis of TOA in this patient. Hydro- or pyosalpinx, a feature of TOA, is not seen with ovarian neoplasms and helps differentiate between the two entities. Pelvic fat stranding and rim-enhancing fluid collection suggest localized peritonitis, a complication of pelvic inflammatory disease.

Teaching Points

▶ TOA formation, pyosalpinx, and peritonitis are complications of pelvic inflammatory disease.

▶ TOA are usually caused by ascending infection from the fallopian tubes but may be secondary to spread of infection from appendicitis, diverticulitis, or other adjacent inflammation.

▶ TOA present with pelvic pain and symptoms of infection but up to 20% may be afebrile without leukocytosis.

▶ On ultrasound, TOA present as complex adnexal structures with ill-defined margins, increased vascularity, thick walls, and internal debris.

Management

▶ Antibiotics; aspiration/drain for large abscesses

Further Reading

Kaakaji Y, Nghiem HV, Nodell C, Winter TC. Sonography of obstetric and gynecologic emergencies: Part II, gynecologic emergencies. *AJR Am J Roentgenol.* 2000;174(3):651–656.

History

▶ 36-year-old woman presents with acute-onset severe right pelvic pain

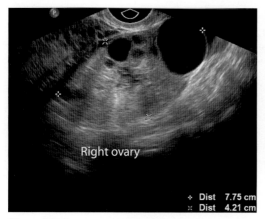

Figure 127.1

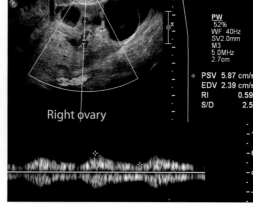

Figure 127.2

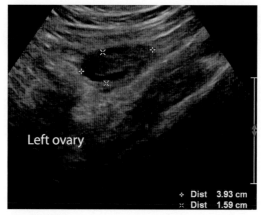

Figure 127.3

Case 127   Ovarian Torsion

Findings

▶ Figure 127.1 is a grayscale ultrasound image showing an abnormal enlarged (measuring up to 7 cm) echogenic right ovary with multiple cysts. Trace-free pelvic fluid is noted.

▶ Color Doppler (Figure 127.2) shows arterial waveform in the right ovary.

▶ Left ovary is normal in size with small follicles (Figure 127.3).

Differential Diagnosis

▶ In this patient with acute-onset right-sided pelvic pain, demonstration of unilateral ovarian enlargement is very concerning for ovarian torsion. Although torsion is classically associated with absent ovarian Doppler flow, arterial flow is present in a significant number of patients with torsion and should not preclude the diagnosis in the setting of strong clinical suspicion and ipsilateral ovarian enlargement. A pregnancy test is used to exclude ectopic pregnancy, which can have similar presentation with acute-onset pain, unilateral adnexal mass/enlargement, and free fluid. Ovarian hyperstimulation syndrome also causes ovarian enlargement but is always bilateral.

Teaching Points

▶ Ovarian torsion is a gynecologic emergency secondary to twisting of the ovary on its vascular pedicle, resulting in compromised ovarian blood supply.

▶ Clinical presentation is with abdominal pain, vomiting, leukocytosis, and fever.

▶ Preexisting ovarian lesions (cysts, dermoids) predispose to ovarian torsion and are the underlying cause in the majority of cases.

▶ Infertility treatment and pregnancy are additional risk factors.

▶ Unilateral ovarian enlargement is the most consistent finding in ovarian torsion.

▶ Doppler findings of torsion are inconsistent, and a significant number of patients with torsion (17%–54%) have detectable flow.

▶ Venous flow is usually occluded before arterial flow. Arterial flow may be demonstrated in ovarian torsion, but it is uncommon to have torsion with normal venous flow.

▶ Free pelvic fluid is often present.

Management

▶ Surgical detorsion or excision

Further Reading

Mashiach R, Melamed N, Gilad N, Ben-Shitrit G, Meizner I. Sonographic diagnosis of ovarian torsion: accuracy and predictive factors. *J Ultrasound Med.* 2011;30(9):1205–1210.

Case 128

History

- 35-year-old woman being treated for infertility

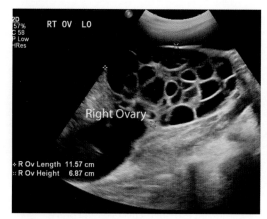

Figure 128.1

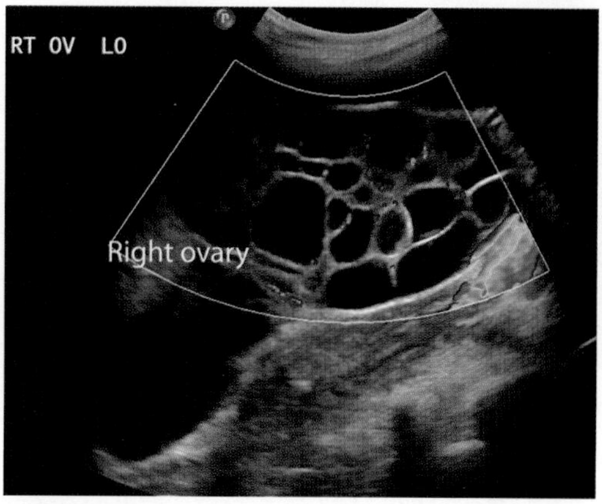

Figure 128.2

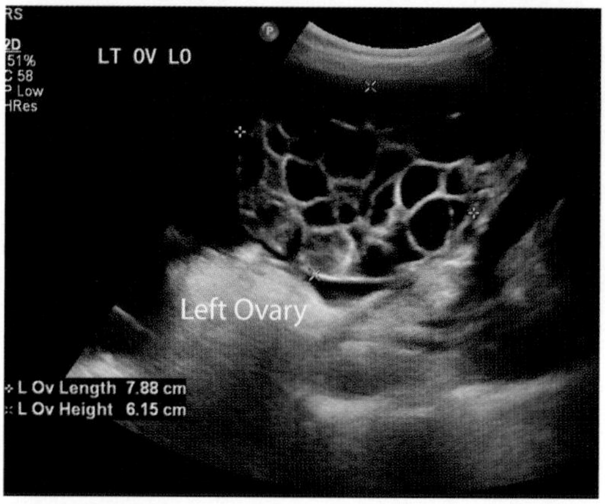

Figure 128.3

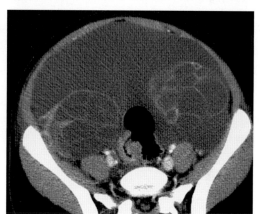

Figure 128.4

Case 128   Ovarian Hyperstimulation Syndrome

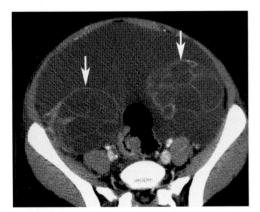

Figure 128.5

Findings

▶ Grayscale and color Doppler images (Figures 128.1 and 128.2) show an extremely enlarged right ovary, measuring up to 11.5 cm. Numerous large cysts/follicles are present throughout the right ovary. Normal ovarian vascularity is present. Large pelvic ascites is noted.

▶ Left ovary is also enlarged and similar in appearance to the right ovary, with numerous cysts/follicles (Figure 128.3).

▶ Contrast CT (Figure 128.4) demonstrates massively enlarged ovaries containing numerous large cysts and large ascites (arrows in Figure 128.5).

Differential Diagnosis

▶ Massive ovarian enlargement with ascites can be due to tosion, tumor, or hyperstimulation. Ovarian torsion can be excluded as it is a unilateral condition. Secondary (Kruckenberg) and, less commonly, primary ovarian tumors can be bilateral and multicystic, but they usually have a nodular soft tissue component. Innumerable ovarian cysts, as noted here, are more consistent with enlarged physiologic follicles than cystic ovarian neoplasm. Echogenic soft tissue between the cysts has the appearance of ovarian stroma and not tumor nodularity. In a patient undergoing treatment for infertility, bilateral massive enlargement of ovaries with numerous variable-sized cysts and ascites is characteristic of ovarian hyperstimulation syndrome.

Teaching Points

▶ Ovarian hyperstimulation is a rare, life-threatening condition secondary to hormonal overstimulation by gonadotrophins.

▶ It is a complication of ovulation induction but rarely occurs spontaneously due to endogenous hormone production.

▶ Clinical presentation is with pain, abdominal distention, nausea, and vomiting.

▶ Ovarian hyperstimulation causes enlargement of follicular cysts and fluid shift, resulting in ascites, plural effusion, hemoconcentration, and oliguria.

▶ On cross-sectional imaging, the central ovarian stroma surrounded by numerous cysts with thin intervening septa has been described as having "spoke-wheel" appearance.

▶ Appropriate clinical setting and imaging features help differentiate ovarian hyperstimulation syndrome from ovarian tumors, preventing unnecessary surgery.

Management

▶ Supportive with discontinuation of infertility stimulants

Further Reading

Baron KT, Babagbemi KT, Arleo EK, Asrani AV, Troiano RN. Emergent complications of assisted reproduction: expecting the unexpected. *Radiographics*. 2013;33(1):229–244.

Case 129

History

- 25-year-old woman with hirsutism, obesity, and oligomenorrhea

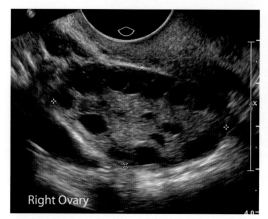

Figure 129.1

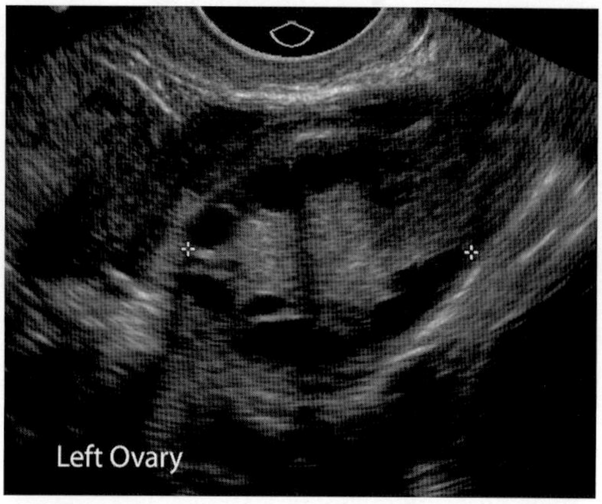

Figure 129.2

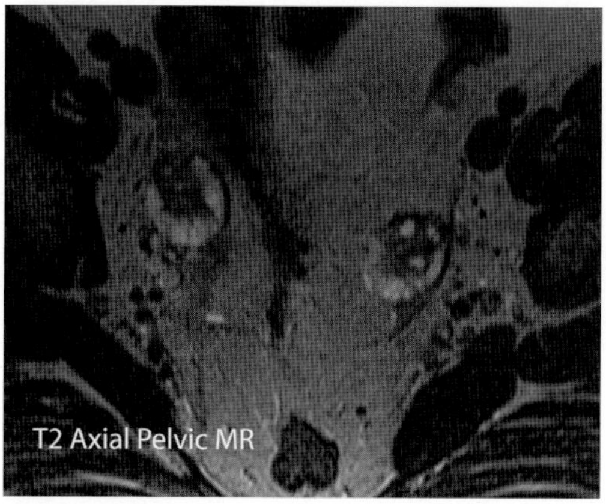

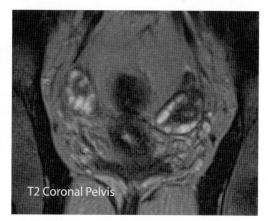

Figure 129.3

Figure 129.4

Case 129 Polycystic Ovarian Syndrome

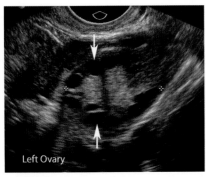

Figure 129.5

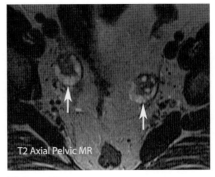

Figure 129.6

Findings

▶ Grayscale ultrasound images of both ovaries (Figures 129.1 and 129.2) show bilateral multiple (at least 12) small (2–8 mm) predominantly peripheral follicles (arrows in Figure 129.5) with central echogenic stroma, giving a string-of-pearls appearance. The calculated volume of the right and left ovary is 13 cc and 14 cc, respectively (not shown).

▶ Axial and coronal T2-weighted MR images (Figures 129.3 and 129.4) show numerous small peripheral follicles (arrows in Figure 129.6).

Differential Diagnosis

▶ Imaging was performed to evaluate the adnexa for presence of polycystic ovaries in view of the hormonal abnormalities. Current ultrasound criteria for identifying polycystic ovaries are ovarian volume >10 cc and presence of at least 12 small (2–8 mm) follicles in each ovary. This patient meets ultrasound criteria for polycystic ovaries. Presence of polycystic ovaries does not establish the diagnosis of polycystic ovarian syndrome (PCOS), which depends on the presence of hyperandrogenism and ovarian dysfunction in addition to polycystic ovaries.

Teaching Points

▶ PCOS is the most common endocrine disorder in women of reproductive age.
▶ Stein Leventhal syndrome is a combination of amenorrhea, obesity, and masculinizing symptoms.
▶ PCOS results due to hypersecretion of androgens, ovulatory dysfunction, and insulin resistance.
▶ A dominant follicle does not develop in PCOS, resulting in multiple 2- to 8-mm follicles.
▶ Previously described ultrasound findings of echogenic stroma and peripheral arrangement of follicles are not required for diagnosis of polycystic ovaries by current criteria.
▶ Polycystic ovaries, as seen on ultrasound, are present in 23% of women of reproductive age. These findings are nonspecific and, in absence of ovulatory dysfunction or hyperandrogenism, do not represent PCOS.
▶ Imaging reports for patients with suspected PCOS should include size and volume of each ovary, number of follicles, and size of the largest follicle.

Management

▶ Pharmacologic treatment

Further Reading
Lee TT, Rausch ME. Polycystic ovarian syndrome: role of imaging in diagnosis. *Radiographics*. 2012;32(6):1643–1657.

Index of Cases

Index